T0276203

Food Fraud

Food Fraud

Food Fraud

Dr. John M. Ryan
Ryan Systems, Inc. Palm Bay,
FL, USA

AMSTERDAM • BOSTON • HEIDELBERG • LONDON
NEW YORK • OXFORD • PARIS • SAN DIEGO
SAN FRANCISCO • SINGAPORE • SYDNEY • TOKYO

Academic Press is an imprint of Elsevier

Academic Press is an imprint of Elsevier
125, London Wall, EC2Y 5AS.
525 B Street, Suite 1800, San Diego, CA 92101-4495, USA
225 Wyman Street, Waltham, MA 02451, USA
The Boulevard, Langford Lane, Kidlington, Oxford OX5 1GB, UK

Notices
Knowledge and best practice in this field are constantly changing. As new research and experience broaden our understanding, changes in research methods or professional practices, may become necessary.

Practitioners and researchers must always rely on their own experience and knowledge in evaluating and using any information or methods described herein. In using such information or methods they should be mindful of their own safety and the safety of others, including parties for whom they have a professional responsibility.

To the fullest extent of the law, neither the Publisher nor the authors, contributors, or editors, assume any liability for any injury and/or damage to persons or property as a matter of products liability, negligence or otherwise, or from any use or operation of any methods, products, instructions, or ideas contained in the material herein.

ISBN: 978-0-12-803393-7

Library of Congress Cataloging-in-Publication Data
A catalog record for this book is available from the Library of Congress

British Library Cataloguing-in-Publication Data
A catalogue record for this book is available from the British Library

For Information on all Academic Press publications
visit our website at http://store.elsevier.com/

Working together
to grow libraries in
developing countries

www.elsevier.com • www.bookaid.org

CONTENTS

INTRODUCTION

Assume you are in the year 2050. In that year, food fraud might not exist. The technology to identify, the laws governing, and the industries involved might all have coordinated through time to control food fraud issues.

Today is 2016. Investigations into and solutions capable of identifying and eliminating food fraud are in their infancy. Today's food supply chain practices create illusions in the minds of consumers.

Adequate traceability, technology, laws, supply chain cooperation, and other factors needed to tackle and control food fraud do not currently exist. The abilities of international communities to identify and eliminate food fraud are, today, poorly defined, uncoordinated, or nonexistent.

International governments, food communities, supply chains, and consumers are relatively immature when it comes to identifying and eliminating what we have yet to legally define as food fraud. Laws, detection technologies, attitudes, and prosecution exist in a piecemeal manner. As the world's population continues to grow, food import, and export demands continue to complicate any government's ability to control food safety and quality and fraudulent practices. As supply chains lengthen, the opportunity to commit food fraud expands as well.

But today's food fraud and international trade situations raise some questions. Is food fraud really a big enough issue to worry about? With the international food fraud annual cost estimated at $10−15 billion, it seems to be a relatively minor concern. Is the low estimated cost why governments aren't responding at a faster rate to establish laws, controls, and enforcement? Yes, there are public food fraud disclosures that tend to upset different segments of society (e.g., horse meat and honey), but other than the daily news, do consumers care? If consumers are rarely concerned, why should the food industry or governments respond? Furthermore, if consumers do care, how does the food industry approach this dilemma?

Many options are open. Ignoring the problem, pretending to take action, watching market response, and working to prevent the problem are all options and represent different paths for different food suppliers.

There are untold and as yet undefined ways to conduct food fraud. Intentionally or not, under today's common food practices or not, our current food production, distribution, and transportation practices are all in line for investigation and prosecution under related food laws. Governments and enforcement agencies are prone to prosecute under any law within their control and this means that without adequate food fraud control laws, they will find a way to prosecute the guilty.

There are many definitions currently in use for "food fraud" but most governments have yet to provide a legal definition. Enforcement and prosecution by any single or multiple governmental entities currently tend to rely on other more established definitions for food safety, adulteration, and the like when attempting to put blame where it belongs.

Confusion reigns over some seemingly conflicting concepts such as "intentional," "for economic gain," and "economically motivated adulteration." Questions are quick to arise. For instance, if a packing house intentionally cuts corners and does not install adequate sanitation and contamination controls over the packing operation due to costs and consumers later become ill due to the adulteration of the food product, can this situation be prosecuted under "economically motivated adulteration" definitions?

Some of the definitions noted in this book are quite narrow in scope while others are broad enough to include all aspects of the food supply chain from harvest through delivery to restaurants, retail outlets, and consumers.

Some individuals and groups are focused on defining food fraud as the "substitution of one ingredient for another" in order to focus prosecution of food fraud more clearly on issues related to ingredients. Incidents such as the European fiasco over the substitution of horse meat for beef while the product was sold as beef or the substitution of cheaper types of fish under labels that inaccurately named the type of fish bring the substitution issue into the realm of mislabeling and economically motivated.

Wikipedia defines fraud as the "deliberate deception to secure unfair or unlawful gain. Fraud is both a civil wrong (i.e., a fraud victim may sue the fraud perpetrator to avoid the fraud and/or recover monetary compensation) and a criminal wrong (i.e., a fraud perpetrator may be prosecuted and imprisoned by governmental authorities)." Webster's dictionary, in part, defines fraud as "intentional perversion of truth in order to induce another to part with something or to surrender a legal right" and "an act of deceiving or misrepresenting" [1].

It seems that in order to deal with what is becoming known as "food fraud" whether or not criminal prosecution is in order, means that a broad understanding of the many more potential types of food fraud need to be looked at and discussed.

Most types of food have been identified as having been somehow fraudulently presented, usually through substitution of ingredients. Some food fraud cases have received significant attention and criminal investigations depending on the degree and type of publicity each has received. Other food fraud cases receive scant attention and many more go unidentified.

In an era when food safety laws are undergoing significant updating and upgrading due to increased international trade, the opportunities for food fraud, in any of its many forms, continue to be found throughout the entire food chain and in any type of food. With food suppliers under constant pressure to reduce costs and deliver on-time, intentional, unintentional, harmful to humans or animals or not, economically motivated or not, adulterated or not, the ingredient approach to food fraud and the perception of what food fraud is and what food fraud is becoming needs to be, like the expanding food supply chain, more of a world view that encompasses more of the options open to questionable practices and suppliers.

As the price of food continues to go up and consumers react by shopping elsewhere or when a recession hits, companies will look for ways to cut costs. When a chief executive issues an order to tighten budgets and cut costs, the strategy for cutting costs may be left to lower level management and further interpreted by all personnel. Cutting costs can mean eliminating refrigeration, using dirty packaging, scrapping the traceability program, reducing training budgets, laying off personnel, using cheaper packaging that outgasses during microwaving, elimination of package sanitation controls, or buying from cheaper or unknown suppliers. Such cost cutting strategies open the door to what may be determined to be economically motivated adulteration. The danger lies in reducing costs that generally focus on longer term strategies designed to reduce risk and prevent problems.

In today's food safety world, tier 1 customers almost universally require some type of food safety certification on the part of their suppliers. Customers generally specify which certification is required and from which company. Suppliers with multiple customers are often forced to attain certification from multiple certification bodies. Over the past dozen years or so, more and more audit groups have developed standards to which the supplier is expected to comply. Audits that cover reviews of the supplier's documentation and record keeping system are conducted at the supplier, a score is established and the supplier receiver (or fails) certification.

To some extent, a conflict of interest exists within the food safety audit process. Audit groups do not want to lose customers. If audits are too tough, it is likely that the supplier will find another auditor or audit group who is not so tough thus cutting the auditing agency out of income received from the supplier. Audits are generally based on visual inspection and review of documentation. They generally require few if any subjective laboratory (hard data) results and, when they do, the supplier may only lose a few points out of hundreds of possible points. A producer may pass a food safety audit even though the water being used to irrigate the crop has been shown by lab tests to be contaminated.

Additionally, audit standards used by auditors often contain subjective words like "adequate," "sufficiently," and "properly" leaving the pass/fail decision up to the auditor. Of equal importance is the fact that there may be no repeatability competency for a single auditor (gives the same score for the same operation under the same conditions) or reliability between auditors (give the same score regardless of the auditor used).

The potential for conflict of interest, subjective observations, lack of dependence on lab data, and lack of auditor repeatability and reliability open the door to audit fraud. It costs money to put together a competent and fair audit system and it costs the supplier money to undergo and pass objective and tightened scrutiny. The food and audit industries continue to resist what are perceived as undue costs in spite of the fact that some companies have soared to high food safety scores only to later be prosecuted for food safety violations [2,3].

Changing the food safety audit system so it is more in line with governmental outbreak audits (sample and lab based results), scientifically sound, fair, and inclusive of food fraud considerations is taboo across the supply chain, due to the potential for negative lab results and for economic reasons. Continuing to rely on such inadequate audit systems for economic reasons while presenting them to the public as a preventive solution opens the door to food fraud at the highest and most sophisticated levels.

Food fraud is not new but with ever improving identification, reporting, and an improving focus by suppliers, better understanding and improved solutions are on the horizon. With more attention comes more data and more analysis. While current trends in food fraud appear to be on the rise, improved detection, reporting, and prosecution all contribute to what seems to be increased food fraud but what may really be the result of an increased focus on the food fraud problem.

Meanwhile, the Grocery Manufacturer's Association's "Consumer Product Fraud Deterrence and Detection" publication of 2010, stated that food fraud continues to be a $10−15 billion annual problem in the US alone. Furthermore, the association calls for the collaboration and action of all supply chain members to work to prevent food fraud [4].

CHAPTER 1

Background

How does a company know what it buys and sells are authentic? How do companies know if the product or content of the food your company paid for has not been intentionally falsified or mislabeled? What practices are considered normal operational procedures in today's food world and provide a basis for defrauding companies and consumers? How can a company protect consumers or their customers when their own company is highly exposed? How can consumers know that what they buy is the product they intended to buy?

Why do some people and companies commit food fraud? One must consider perpetrators to be basically dishonest and to feel that they will not get caught. In other words, the money they make or save is expected by them to exceed the probability that their product will cause problems or will be found out. In some cases, the amount of money to be made significantly exceeds the costs associated with fines.

Frequently a company has no way of knowing whether or not what they buy or sell is fraudulent or includes fraudulent contents. This brings up the question of who is liable for what any company sells. Product liability as established under FDA current good manufacturing practices (cGMP) make the food manufacturer liable for the production, packaging, labeling, and holding of foods. This makes the manufacturer responsible for ensuring that the ingredients used in production meet current good manufacturing requirements. Along with this is a requirement for manufacturers to assure that the key ingredients used in food production are as required and reported. This verification requirement establishes the food manufacturer as liable for their products.

The thinking behind this is simple. Any manufacturer (food or otherwise) is, according to normal quality requirements, responsible for the qualification and certification of all suppliers. Supplier qualification is a process that normally requires a company to visit and provide due diligence over the supplier, its processes, and ingredients prior

Food Fraud. DOI: http://dx.doi.org/10.1016/B978-0-12-803393-7.00001-9

to using that supplier. Certification generally requires that the supplier in question must have established quality, sanitation, and other controls specified by the company in question. Once a supplier is qualified and certified, the hiring company then assumes some part of the liability for the supplier's actions and products.

Horse meat labeled as beef in Europe, unlabeled GMO (genetically modified organisms) products, and literally hundreds of other foods and liquors are intentionally modified or mislabeled for economic reasons. In the United States and many other countries, new laws are being written and enacted to protect, not only the food supply chain, but consumers from fraudulent practices.

Under the United States Food and Drug Administration (FDA) food fraud is defined as the "Fraudulent, intentional substitution or addition of a substance in a product for the purpose of increasing the apparent value of the product or reducing the cost of its production, i.e., for economic gain." However, in the United States, no single federal agency and no single US law or statute directly addresses food fraud or "economically motivated adulteration" of food and food ingredients.

In a January 2014 report by Renee Johnson entitled "Economically Motivated Adulteration" of Food and Food Ingredients, Renee summarizes data from the United States Pharmacopeial (USP) Convention Food Fraud Database database. When summarized, oils, milk, juices, spices, and sweeteners account for 69% of the reported types between the years of 1980 and 2010, while natural flavors, spices, seafood, and grains/cereals headed the list of food ingredient fraudulent cases. In her report, substitution of ingredients account for 65% of the economically motivated incidents for the same period. Most of these food fraud findings came from production in the United States (29.8%), China (13.6%), and India (12.6%) [5].

1.1 RISK

There are a number of potential food fraud risk raising opportunities that might be considered. Some of these risk opportunities include products using high value ingredients, ingredients that are easy to disguise, hard to see or test for, bulk products, globalization and trade, supply chains that are not vertically integrated (known suppliers, carriers, etc.), suppliers without cGMP supplier certification and those with no incoming testing programs. Suppliers with previously reported poor food safety, poor food quality, or poor manufacturing processes represent another set of high risk producers and processors. Many opportunists simply feel that the likelihood of being caught is so low that it is worth their personal risk to pursue fraudulent opportunities. In other words, the financial rewards exceed the risk of being caught and successfully prosecuted.

As international food trade increases, food processors, distributors, and consumers are purchasing more and more food from foreign countries often with inadequate oversight or control over what is coming across borders and into supermarkets, restaurants, and refrigerators. With new international laws focused on bringing food importers into the receiving country's compliance certification programs, and with each country's inability to provide enforcement coverage at ports, opportunities to slip fraudulent foods across borders increase. To a great extent, this import problem becomes one of risk and how one assesses risk.

Risk is often estimated as the probability of something happening and that probability is often difficult to assess for many reasons. Developing preventive strategies focused on reducing risk is the task of all food suppliers. But preventing fraudulent product from entering the food chain requires the development of certification programs and, sometimes, strenuous testing technologies and strategies to keep fraudulent food products out of the supply chain. As of today, hindsight rules the development of testing capable of detecting fraudulent ingredients or products. New tests and the application of older test technologies are generally developed after public exposure of fraudulent activities. While many consider product and ingredient testing to prevent human illness, food fraud, and death, testing, in terms of quality control concepts, is not a preventive activity. Incoming testing causes companies to expend millions of dollars in order to assure that their often uncertified suppliers are not cheating.

The Grocery Manufacturer's Association (GMA), as an example, recommends an incoming test followed by rejection and return of the product for a lack of conformance to requirements. However, the strategy is greatly weakened because the choice of testing and analysis is based greatly on previous history of the product and attempted adulterant.

A farmer may assess the type of risk planting and harvesting a particular product based on recall and CODEX data. But when that product becomes an ingredient in a more complex processing operation, the burden of risk assessment is often passed on to the processor.

With international trade over long distances currently without international rules, agreements and enforcement make overall risk in food trade difficult to estimate and, more importantly, difficult to prevent and control.

Some facts remain. Many variables come into play when forces in favor of informed decision making by consumers comes up against governments, companies, or individuals with something to hide that will impact their marketing goals. While the vast majority of food fraud incidents do not pose a public health risk, most of those people or companies committing food fraud want to avoid detection and go to great lengths to do so. The problem is compounded because internationally it is not known how widespread food fraud is nor are there acceptable legal definitions established.

Taken together, the thinking that food fraud incidents that do not pose a public health risk (e.g., horse meat in lieu of beef) opens a Pandora's box involving legislation, legislators, campaign funding, consumer advocates, and large corporations that might influence law makers decision making when it comes to establishing more rigid label requirements. Many companies may claim that significant label omissions are valid (e.g., GMO) in light of a lack of scientific evidence supporting hypotheses that such ingredient changes might be harmful.

The thinking that whether or not a product is intended to cause harm or not intended to cause harm to humans continues to muddy the food fraud waters. While arguments over GMO and product labeling requirements continue to fan food fraud flames, the long term human impact of products and ingredients is rarely studied.

In many cases, the lack of scientific evidence against a particular ingredient or practice is merely a lack of the impact that new ingredients might have over two or three generations of consumers. Longitudinal studies that cover a generation of use are generally lacking, leaving the public afraid of the consequences that new or different ingredients might have on their health. Genetically modified corn and soy are good examples of such scenarios but only represent the tip of the iceberg when it comes to a lack of labeling requirements and the battles that ensue. Lobbyists hired by many companies continue to influence decision makers at governmental levels in an effort to eliminate the enactment of labeling requirements that provide informed decision making.

When governmental agencies such as the FDA decide that some product or practice is generally regarded as safe (GRAS), it should be remembered that the FDA does not do the testing of the product or process. Usually the product manufacturer is responsible for designing and carrying out research, under FDA guidance, that is scientifically sound and intended to fulfill substantial evidence regarding whether or not a particular practice or product is safe for its intended use. While GMO ingredients are GRAS based on the short term studies provided by the companies that develop and market GMO products, such label omissions deprive the consumer of information relevant to the purchase and deny the idea that GMO ingredients might later (through longitudinal studies) be classified as adulterants. Clearly, the use of GMO ingredients and products are not intended to cause human harm. But scientific manipulation, lobbying and the other strategies that might be employed to attain GRAS status are in pursuit of economic gain.

Do such practices place GMO products in the fraudulent category as defined by the FDA in 2009

Fraudulent, intentional substitution or addition of a substance in a product for the purpose of increasing the apparent value of the product or reducing the cost of its production, i.e., for economic gain [6].

Such labeling dilemmas, to some extent, exacerbate the ability to clearly define food fraud. Is food fraud intentional adulteration of food? Is food fraud intended to "obtain economic gain and not cause public health harm although public health harm may occur"? Is food fraud a food safety issue? Should it come under food safety rules?

This brief book will explore the current state of supply chain food fraud, the laws being enacted to try to control it and the level of fraud currently in operation. In the European Union (EU) changes to the food safety laws are underway. In the United States, the FDA has established new "intentional adulteration" and "economically motivated adulteration" rules based on the Food Safety Modernization Act (FSMA) and, based on international acknowledgment of the problem, other countries are enhancing their own import controls over illegal replacements.

1.2 PREVENTION VERSUS CORRECTIVE ACTION

In many industries the term "corrective action" is often confused with preventive concepts. This is certainly the case within the food industries. Corrective action does not reduce risk and does not involve causal analysis but rather is usually an attempt to reduce the likelihood of further impact for some problem that was not originally prevented. In many industries, corrective action is associated with the recall, rework, disposal, separation, isolation, removal, or return of some product that has intentionally or accidentally escaped into the trade and consumer arenas. Corrective action practices generally involve the formation of some type of committee or group to decide how to lessen the public impact of the escape and to identify where the escaped product is, herd the product into isolation and then to determine the escaped product's fate. In some industries, the corrective action group or team is called a "material review board" that consists of varying members from throughout the organization's functional structure. The need is for financial, quality, safety, operations, engineering, and other personnel to collectively determine how to reduce the impact of the escape on the organization in question.

Escaped (or recalled) product means that the organization in question either intentionally allowed the escape in hopes that it would not be discovered, or accidentally, through poor controls, missed some critical step in their processes that was, or should have been, designed to eliminate the possibility of such escapes. Escapes that are identified and publicly reported represent the most expensive failure a company or organization can experience due to the recall costs, damage to the brand name, law suits, loss of customers, and associated enforcement and prosecution.

From a quality control perspective, food escapes to a recall situation are called external failures. Without adequate supply chain of custody traceability systems in place, the time period between escape and control becomes unacceptable when it comes to protecting innocent companies and consumers. Without supply chain of custody traceability systems in place, intentional and unintentional fraudsters continue to operate behind curtains of illusion and magic.

Once the escape has come under control, the organizational challenge becomes one of determining what caused the escape. The determination of cause is often complicated, far reaching, time consuming, and expensive but generally not considered as expensive as costs associated with the external failure. The purpose of causal analysis is to pinpoint changes the organization must make in order to eliminate the possibility that the cause can recur. The change process often requires organizations to upgrade operational and quality procedures, attitudes, or personnel. A good causal analysis program often reduces finger pointing and improper damage control practices.

CHAPTER 2

Some Food Fraud Laws

With ever expanding food import and distribution networks, many food supply companies are experiencing previously unheard of challenges. Knowing the source and content of perishable and processed foods becomes somewhat impossible without more modern technological and food safety solutions. Newly evolving solutions such as traceability, test, audit, and certification are, today, incapable of providing the level of protection theoretically possible in modern societies.

Added to food suppliers' challenges are consumers who are becoming more and more aware of the potential impact that unhealthy diets, pesticides, poor labeling, fraudulent food, and food from unknown sources may have on them and their families. Daily news headlines blast details of contaminated foods, human illness, death, economically motivated food adulteration, and out-and-out fraud. All of this sets the food industry into occasional spins that cost producers, shippers, distributors, carriers, retailers, restaurants, and processors millions upon millions of dollars.

When focusing on food fraud, there are quite a number of food fraud issues that need to be considered. These include:

- Economically Motivated Adulteration (EMA)
- US and other country laws designed to control food fraud
- Labeling omissions
- Unstandardized, haphazard traceability systems
- Packaging
- Genetically Modified Organisms (GMO)
- The products themselves: Fish, horsemeat, honey, flavoring, colors, oils, sweeteners, juices, dairy, liquors, and many more
- Detection testing technologies
- Adulteration, substitution, tampering, and counterfeiting
- Reporting food fraud
- Prevention

Food Fraud. DOI: http://dx.doi.org/10.1016/B978-0-12-803393-7.00002-0

There are as many ways to conduct food fraud as there are products involved: Substituting one ingredient for another, adding ice and water to increase weight, adding salt, providing false vitamin claims, counterfeiting, adding drugs to food (especially animal feeds), flame retardants in juices, misleading labels, and offering "blends" in lieu of "100% pure" are only a few.

As food fraud issues continue to be exposed, more and more research is being conducted to determine the extent to which the public is exposed to food fraud. In the UK, The Guardian reported in February of 2014 that testing of meat products showed that they were found to contain what is referred to as meat emulsion (or pink slime in the United States). Also, many other misleading, unlabeled or mysterious additives and substitutes were discovered through testing of over 900 products. Over one-third of the products tested failed label comparison and ingredient tests [7].

2.1 DEFINING FOOD FRAUD IN THE EUROPEAN UNION

The Food Standards Agency headquartered in London, England defines food fraud as "Food fraud is committed when food is deliberately placed on the market, for financial gain, with the intention of deceiving the consumer" which includes the sale of any unfit and potential harmful food, mislabeling, product or ingredient substitution, and making false statements. The agency recommends whistle blowing and other means of reporting food fraud to their database. They also provide money for enforcement and an advisory unit for local authorities [8].

The European Union, being comprised of numerous countries with varied laws, has at its core a collective consideration for the free movement of food throughout the European community and protection of citizenry through standardized agreement on general food safety and quality requirements. Although without a firm definition of food fraud, the European Parliament and of the Council of January 28, 2002 provides guidance under Article 8 in Regulation (EC) No 178/2002

Article 8
Protection of consumers' interests

1. *Food law shall aim at the protection of the interests of consumers and shall provide a basis for consumers to make informed choices in relation to the foods they consume. It shall aim at the prevention of:*
   a. *fraudulent or deceptive practices;*
   b. *the adulteration of food; and*
   c. *any other practices which may mislead the consumer [9].*

2.2 DEFINING FOOD FRAUD IN THE UNITED STATES

On April 30, 2011, John Spink and Douglas Moyer at Michigan State University defined food fraud as part of a grant from the National Center for Food Protection and Defense. Spinks and Moyer are perhaps the preeminent experts in food fraud and specialize in linking food fraud to criminology in an effort to provide preventive mechanisms.

Food fraud is a collective term used to encompass the deliberate and intentional substitution, addition, tampering, or misrepresentation of food, food ingredients, or food packaging; or false or misleading statements made about a product, for economic gain [10].

Their definition is an expansion of the Food and Drug Administration (FDA) EMA definition.

In "Food Fraud and Economically Motivated Adulteration of Food and Food Ingredients" (January 10, 2014) Renee Johnson, a specialist in agricultural policy, defines food fraud as "the act of defrauding buyers of food or ingredients for economic gain." She notes that the US has no legal definition of either food fraud or EMA [6].

The United States Department of Agriculture (USDA), Food and Drug Administration, Center for Disease Control, US Customs, Homeland Security, and a myriad of other federal, state and local agencies (Table 2.1) have, under newly combined US federal laws and rules, begin to work together as they grope for enforcement solutions. The US Congress passed the Food Safety Modernization Act (FSMA) that has been continuously ensnarled in bureaucracy for years while the food supply chain continues to ask for firm direction and answers. Meanwhile, the larger food supply chain members actively lobby to further complicate and delay finalization of FSMA rules. The legal concern is focused on enforcement which is a primary focus of federal, state, and local agencies while businesses focus on costs and having to change their processes.

While some in the Federal government see a need for a unified single food safety organization, resistance is high for those wanting to protect their own authority and position. For instance while the FDA is responsible for food (but not meat), dietary supplements, bottled water, seafood, wild game, and eggs in the shell, the USDA is responsible for the grading of raw fruit and vegetables, meat, poultry, egg processing and grading, and certifying organic production. The National Oceanic and Atmospheric Administration grades fish and seafood and the EPA is responsible for drinking water and pesticide

Table 2.1 FDA Allies
Centers for Disease Control and Prevention (CDC)
Environmental Protection Agency (EPA)—activities related to establishing priorities and addressing other issues related to residues of animal drugs and pesticides in food animals, detecting illegal residues, and taking regulatory action against violators
US Department of Agriculture, Food Safety Inspection Service (FSIS)—meat, poultry, and processed eggs
US Department of Agriculture, Agricultural Marketing Service (AMS)—egg shell safety
U.S. Department of Agriculture, Foreign Agricultural Service (FAS)—coordinate future activities and approaches to selected food safety issues facing developing countries and emerging markets
US Department of Agriculture, Food and Nutrition Service (FNS)—FDA-regulated products distributed via domestic nutrition assistance programs administered by FNS. Examples of such programs include the National School Lunch Program and Emergency Food Assistance Program
US Department of Homeland Security (DHS)—DHS personnel formally commissioned and specially trained to conduct cargo and other examinations of FDA-regulated articles. CBP personnel have authority to hold suspect shipments for further examination and sampling
US Department of Commerce, National Oceanic and Atmospheric Administration, National Marine Fisheries Service (NMFS)—Seafood—NMFS inspects 20% of seafood consumed in the United States
US Department of Defense (DOD)—information sharing
US Department of Labor, Occupational Safety and Health Administration (OSHA)
Federal Trade Commission (FTC)

residues. The Department of Justice covers law enforcement, the Federal Trade Commission (FTC) covers advertising, and the Alcohol and Tobacco Tax and Trade Bureau (TTB) covers alcohol. Customs and Border Protection (CBP) handles enforcement and referral for imported goods. And, the DHS has the authority to ensure the safety and security of imported food. One would have to wonder who covers food fraud.

Through such collective cooperation, laws enacted on behalf of one governmental organization are used to support other governmental enforcement efforts. Such cooperation further extends each organization's reach while reducing overall governmental costs. However, in the United States, no single federal agency and no single US law or statute directly addresses food fraud or "economically motivated adulteration" of food and food ingredients.

As a matter of fact, the FDA exempts the following when it comes to intentional adulteration rules:

- companies with less than $10,000,000 in total annual sales of food, adjusted for inflation

- holding of food, except the holding of food in liquid storage tanks
- packing, repacking, labeling, or relabeling of food where the container that directly contacts the food remains intact
- activities of a facility that are subject to Standards for Produce Safety
- alcoholic beverages at a facility that meets certain conditions
- manufacturing, processing, packing, or holding of food for animals other than man [13]

The head of the FDA's efforts to develop and implement the FSMA, Michael R. Taylor, Deputy Commissioner for Foods, US Food and Drug Administration, puts the responsibility for safe food clearly on the heads of every member of the food industry. He states, "stated in the simplest terms, the recognized solution to the problem of foodborne illness is a comprehensive prevention strategy that involves all participants in the food system, domestic and foreign, doing their part to minimize the likelihood of harmful contamination. And that is the strategy mandated by FSMA. It is not a strategy that assumes we can achieve a zero-risk food supply, but it is a strategy grounded in the conviction that we can better protect consumers and the economic vigor of the food system if everyone involved implements reasonably available measures to reduce risk."[1]

"The FSMA strategy recognizes that the food industry has the primary responsibility and capacity to produce safe food, but it calls for a new definition of public and private roles on food safety and a modern new framework for regulatory oversight, integration of government food safety efforts, and public-private collaboration."

The FDA has clearly established their enforcement strategy by placing primary responsibility on all members of the food industry. Further, under Title I, Improving capacity to prevent food safety problems (Section 101, Inspection of Records), it establishes the agency's rights and responsibilities to have "access to and copy all records" related to the prevention of food safety problems:

(1) Adulterated food.-- Use of or exposure to food of concern. If the Secretary believes that there is a reasonable probability that the use of or

---

[1]http://www.fda.gov/Food/GuidanceRegulation/FSMA/ucm319053.htm 2012. FDA Science Writers Symposium Silver Spring, MD September 11, 2012. As prepared for delivery by Michael R. Taylor Deputy Commissioner for Foods U.S. Food and Drug Administration.

exposure to an article of food, and any other article of food that the Secretary reasonably believes is likely to be affected in a similar manner, will cause serious adverse health consequences or death to humans or animals, each person (excluding farms and restaurants) who manufactures, processes, packs, distributes, receives, holds, or imports such article shall, at the request of an officer or employee duly designated by the Secretary, permit such officer or employee, upon presentation of appropriate credentials and a written notice to such person, at reasonable times and within reasonable limits and in a reasonable manner, to have access to and copy all records relating to such article and to any other article of food that the Secretary reasonably believes is likely to be affected in a similar manner, that are needed to assist the Secretary in determining whether there is a reasonable probability that the use of or exposure to the food will cause serious adverse health consequences or death to humans or animals. "(3) Application.--The requirement under paragraphs (1) and (2) applies to all records relating to the manufacture, processing, packing, distribution, receipt, holding, or importation of such article maintained by or on behalf of such person [[Page 124 STAT. 3887]] in any format (including paper and electronic formats) and at any location."

The FDA presents an operational strategy that highlights:

1. The central external force driving change is the dramatic expansion in the global scale and complexity of the food system
2. Reducing the risk of preventable foodborne illness in today's global food system
3. FDA's primary focus will be on improved public health outcomes
4. Working in partnership to create an integrated global food safety network
5. Use an expanded oversight tool kit that includes both traditional and new tools
6. Implementing the strategic and risk-based industry oversight framework that is at the heart of FSMA (Enforcement—Inspection & Compliance, Administrative Compliance Tools, Judicial Enforcement Tools)
7. Developing strategies, capacity building, training, and operational plans.

Under the FSMA, seven key sets of proposed rules have been published by the FDA. These include:

1. Standards for the Growing, Harvesting, Packing, and Holding of Produce for Human Consumption

2. Current Good Manufacturing Practice and Hazard Analysis and Risk-Based Preventive Controls for Human Food
3. Accreditation of Third-Party Auditors/Certification Bodies to Conduct Food Safety Audits and to Issue Certifications
4. Food Supplier Verification Programs (FSVP) for Importers of Food for Humans and Animals
5. Current Good Manufacturing Practice and Hazard Analysis and Risk-Based Preventive Controls for Food for Animals
6. Focused Mitigation Strategies to Protect Food Against Intentional Adulteration (includes EMA)
7. Sanitary Transportation of Human and Animal Food

Proposed rule number 6 addresses food fraud. The following Table 2.2 is extracted from Figure 3.1 of the FDA's Focused Mitigation Strategies to Protect Food against Intentional Adulteration (3) [12].

As part of the FSMA, the FDA recommends approaching intentional adulteration in standard terms including:

1. Preparing and implementing a written food defense plan
2. Identifying and implementing focused mitigation strategies at each actionable process step to prevent adulteration at each step

Table 2.2 FDA Summary: Focused Mitigation Strategies to Protect Food against Intentional Adulteration		
Type of Intentional Adulteration	Coverage within Scope of Proposed 21 CFR 121	Brief Rationale, and Relevant Corresponding Section of the Rule [12]
I. Types of Intentional Adulteration Considered in this Proposed Rulemaking		
1. Acts of disgruntled employees, consumers, or competitors intended to attack the reputation of a company, and not to cause public health harm, although public health harm may occur	Not within the scope of intentional adulteration covered under proposed 21 CFR 121	Not considered "high risk" because not intended to cause widespread, significant public health harm. See section IV.E of this document.
2. Economically motivated adulteration (EMA) intended to obtain economic gain, and not to cause public health harm, although public health harm may occur	Not within the scope of intentional adulteration covered under proposed 21 CFR 121	Considering addressing as part of hazard analysis in a preventive controls framework where EMA is "reasonably likely to occur." See section IV.F of this document.
3. Acts intended to cause massive public health harm, including acts of terrorism	Covered within scope, and is the focus of proposed 21 CFR 121	Considered "high risk" because intent of the act is to cause widespread, significant public health harm.

3. Establishing procedures
4. Corrective Action Planning (includes prevention)
5. Verifying that monitoring is being conducted
6. Training Personnel
7. Keeping Records

It seems that regardless of various rules and confusion of whether or not food fraud is included under economically motivated or intentional adulteration rules with exemptions, what the FDA calls "focused mitigation strategies" under the FSMA must be written and followed. These focused mitigation strategies include:

Monitoring
Corrective Action (Prevention)
Verification
Implementation and effectiveness
Reanalysis
Documentation
Training and
Records

That set of strategies illustrates the lack of awareness on the part of FDA food safety officials for what the FDA drug and medical device side has been doing for decades. In a sense, the food side of the FDA continues to befuddle well established quality control practices with new jargon and misdirection as a result of a lack of depth in terms of experience and training within their ranks.

2.3 EXECUTIVE RESPONSIBILITIES AND PROSECUTION: THE PARK DOCTRINE

Over the past few years, peanuts, caramelized apples, expired eggs, and contaminated cantaloupes have all resulted in highly publicized food adulteration criminal prosecution cases. In some instances, the FDA has wrapped its arms around legal precedents under the Office of Criminal Investigations (OCI). The OCI reviews FDA criminal investigation recommendations. In some cases, the Park Doctrine is used by the FDA in prosecutions, especially those classified as food fraud. According to the FDA regulatory procedures manual, "the Park Doctrine, as established by Supreme Court case law, provides that a responsible corporate official can be held liable for a first time misdemeanor (and possible subsequent felony) under the Federal Food, Drug, and Cosmetic Act ('the Act') without proof that the corporate official acted with intent or even negligence, and even if such corporate official did not have any actual knowledge of, or participation in, the specific offense [13]."

The Park Doctrine, in allowing the FDA to prosecute corporate executives, has created a scenario that forces the chief executive to know, be involved in, and take responsibility for food safety through operational reviews and a more hands-on approach.

Most food safety standards and food safety audits today contain a set of management standards and requirements that seek to assure that corporate officers are intimately involved in managing the planned food safety system. Legal professionals are now recommending that food companies establish someone directly responsible for compliance and some type of internal audit/review group be identified who are capable of assuring implementation and compliance with needed procedures. These recommendations represent a basic food safety requirement for food safety certification. Thus, corporate officers can no longer defend themselves by saying they did not know what was going on with regard to food safety, food quality, or food fraud. In other words, not knowing is no longer a defense nor does the corporate structure provide protection in the food fraud arena.

2.4 FDA TIES WITH CUSTOMS AND BORDER PROTECTION AND HOMELAND SECURITY

The reader might recall that earlier a review of the various agencies working in support of FDA enforcement actions was presented (Table 2.1: Allies). On one hand, the dependence on so many agencies for enforcement means that coordination between and among agencies is difficult. On the other hand, the FDA has the opportunity to keep its internal operating costs low while simultaneously expanding its enforcement capabilities.

Alignment with CBP and the DHS allows the FDA to train and hand off some responsibilities for enforcing food import compliance. Transportation of food products by truck or rail across US borders for consumption in the US means that the combined capabilities of the FDA, CBP, and DHS can all be utilized to further control food fraud.

Laws established under CBP and DHS can be coupled with new FDA rules on the transportation of human and animal foods to cover just about all import enforcement available today. Of course, there is still no way that all three agencies can open, inspect, and test products coming into the United States. However, as agency and interagency databases continue to evolve, a food importer's food safety certification status and inspection and compliance history can be reviewed as food is transported to the border and the container or trailer can be side lined if previous histories indicate that the shipment might be of high risk. This means that the high risk companies will more likely be identified and stopped at the borders and held until inspection by one of the three agencies is conducted.

For the shipper, this means longer border crossing delays, potential stops, and perhaps shipment seizures, all resulting in higher costs [14].

2.5 INTRODUCTION OF AN ADULTERATED FOOD INTO INTERSTATE COMMERCE

Along with the lack of a legal definition of food fraud, uncoordinated government enforcement, politics, and the inability to head off fraudulent products through low cost, fast testing, agencies work to prosecute under older, more established laws. The Offices of the United States Attorneys provides the following example prosecuted under interstate commerce.

Sample Indictment: Interstate Shipment of Adulterated Food

1. *Those parts described as Part A* Introduction, *paragraphs 1 through 18 inclusive, of Count 1 of this Indictment are incorporated specifically herein and are alleged as if set forth in full in these Counts.*
2. *On or about the dates listed below, in the Western District of Michigan and elsewhere, the defendants,*

REALGOOD PRODUCTS COMPANY, FEELIN FINE FOODS CORPORATION, XXXXX X. XXXXXX,

with the intent to defraud and mislead, introduced and delivered for introduction, and caused to be introduced and delivered for introduction, into interstate commerce, for delivery from Realgood in Lansing, Michigan, to Feelin Fine in Chicago, Illinois, adulterated foods, to wit: Foods fraudulently labeled as, and otherwise fraudulently represented to be, orange juice from concentrate.

3. *The foods were adulterated within the meaning of the following sec-*
tions of Title 21, United States Code: Section 342(b)(2), in that beet
sugar and syrup containing beet sugar were substituted in part for
orange juice and orange juice concentrate; Section 342(b)(3), in that
citric acid and amino acids were added to those foods to conceal dam-
age and inferiority; and Section 342(b)(4), in that citric acid, amino
acids, and a preservative were added to and mixed and packed with
those foods so as to make them appear better and of greater value
than they were. Each instance listed below is a separate and additional
Count of this Indictment [15].

Wallin and Klarich (attorneys) report under the Federal Food Drug
and Cosmetic Act (21 USC Section 331) that the distribution of
expired food into interstate commerce is a "felony for intent to defraud
by way of misbranding products" if the food is introduced for sale,
delivered, received, or manufactured. They cite mislabeling, packaging
lacking the name/address of the manufacturer, packager or distributor,
inaccurate quantities (weight, measure, count), misleading statements,
and other criteria. They also note that refusal to allow access to
records maintenance of records as well as refusal to allow inspection of
products are violations [16].

In "Food Safety Issues: FDA Judicial Enforcement Actions,"
Emily M. Lanza, Legislative Attorney (Congressional Research
Service), notes that the FDA maintains enforcement authority and
may file an injunction "against an industry participant to stop or prevent a violation of the FFDCA and to halt the flow of violative products in interstate commerce." Further, the FDA has a right of
seizure:

Seizure
The FDA Under Section 304(a)(1) of the FFDCA, the government may seize
an article of food in interstate commerce that is adulterated or misbranded. A
seizure is a civil action used by the federal government when the removal of
adulterated or misbranded goods from interstate commerce is necessary to
reduce consumer accessibility to those goods in order to protect public health.

The seizure must occur when the goods are in interstate commerce or held
for sale after shipment in interstate commerce. The FFDCA broadly defines
interstate commerce as "commerce between any State or Territory and any
place outside thereof." Goods destined for sale in a state other than the place
from which they are shipped qualify as goods in "interstate commerce," even
though they may not have yet physically crossed a boundary. In this context,
courts have also interpreted "interstate commerce" to mean imported foods
held at a port of entry into the United States [17].

2.6 THE POTENTIAL FOR TERRORISM

Although food fraud is commonly defined in a manner that implies the fraudster is economically motivated and has no intent to harm people, the potential for terrorism or intentionally substituting or adding ingredients with the intent to harm people has to be considered. Terrorist food tactics generally fall under food defense considerations but represent the worst type of food fraud activities. The intent to harm is real and can have huge consequences. Even worse, due to the lag between the development of tests and test strategies focused on food fraud and the variety of potential substitutes or added ingredients, opportunities for terrorists to impact thousands of people are literally unlimited.

The terrorist does not necessarily have to come from an organized group but may be a disgruntled employee desiring to destroy an employer's reputation by lacing an avocado shipment with a deadly substance that will go into the soft avocado meat when a knife is used to open the skin.

CHAPTER 3

Food Fraud Through the Supply Chain

Taking a look at Figure 3.1, we can count 17 food transfer points between field harvest and the store shelf for a nonprocessed food. For this illustration, there is movement on a ship between transferring the shipment from the wholesale distributor to the trucked shipping container, dock load, shipping, unload, and a third truck operation to the second distributor.

Viewing the supply chain as a process allows management to define and measure food identity and condition under real-time conditions while storing critical data for future use. The concept of supply chain visibility changes the "one up and one down" approach to one of a chain of custody traceability approach. The shift to the chain of custody perspective is more conducive to food safety and food quality

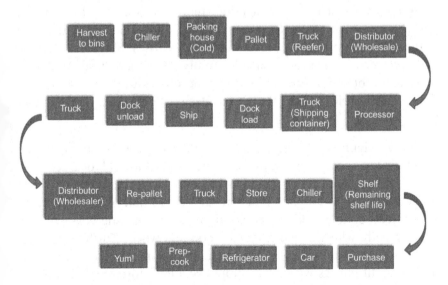

Figure 3.1 Food Supply Chain Example.

Food Fraud. DOI: http://dx.doi.org/10.1016/B978-0-12-803393-7.00003-2

management through all handlers. With today's new technologies, especially traceability technologies, the ability to know the location, identity, and condition of the food throughout the supply chain is available at a reasonable cost. These new technologies provide all supply chain members with real-time visibility. Under newly proposed Food Safety Modernization Act (FSMA) food transportation rules on the sanitary transportation of human and animal foods, the carrier is responsible for assuring that the shipper receives data regarding load temperature maintenance throughout transportation processes.

"One-up and one-down" approaches to traceability generally do not provide such complete data since there is a reliance on cheap data loggers. Data loggers that record temperatures within the trailer compartment are generally either read visually by the receiver or removed from the trailer with data manually downloaded into a computer. From a manpower cost perspective, that is a relatively expensive labor intensive process regardless of the low cost of the data logger itself.

New technologies allow all supply chain members to access and store all temperature data using cell phone technology. The FSMA transportation rules can be easily satisfied by any and all parties using either a cell phone or a tablet that carries a free downloaded app. This means that the location, identity, and condition of the food in the entire supply chain is available to all parties: Shippers, carriers, and receivers. This means that the supply chain is, to a great extent, no longer a bunch of uncoordinated hand-off segments, but an identifiable, recordable process that lends itself to improved management practices.

Supply chain food transportation data can now be stored in the cloud for later access and analysis. In the event of a recall or trace back operation, data that shows exactly when and where the food was at any particular moment provides much advanced and quicker recall control. When questionable food enters the supply chain, investigators can now know exactly who was handling the food and when. Furthermore, the data is, under proposed rules, kept for a minimum period of 1 year thus providing all parties with much more accurate information capable of pinpointing a variety of potential food fraud practices.

When a processing step is added, the supply chain lengthens and provides a significant number of other opportunities for fraud to occur. Processing frequently requires added ingredients which can be purposely substituted for intended ingredients (e.g., melamine for milk). Under current good manufacturing practices in the United States, manufacturers have the responsibility for determining that any claims made about products are substantiated and not false or misleading. Manufacturing practices must ensure that food and dietary supplements are processed to meet quality standards and must include consideration of the design and construction of physical plants, implementing quality control procedures, testing manufactured products and supplements, maintaining records, and handling consumer complaints.

3.1 LABELING

Incorrect, incomplete, and inappropriate labeling is one of the main reasons for food recalls. The recalls are usually conducted due to undisclosed or incorrect ingredients. The FDA provides Guidance for Industry in "A Food Labeling Guide: General Food Labeling Requirements." In addition to label location requirements, the Guide lists certain other requirements for information, statements, type size, and requirements for the manufacturer, packer or distributor name and address [18].

Basic labeling guidance from the guide includes the following label sections:

General Labeling Requirements
• Name of Food
• Juices
• Net Quantity of Contents Statements
• Ingredient Lists
• Nutrition Labeling
• Colors
• Food Allergen Labeling
• Nutrient Declaration
• Products with Separately Packaged Ingredients

The FDA further specifies that ingredients must be listed in descending order of predominance by weight, must include water when added to the product, chemical preservatives, spices, natural and artificial flavors, fat and oil content, trace amounts, vegetable powders, artificial colors, color additives, food additives, allergens, and standards of identity.

Label Formats/Graphics
• General
• Specific Label Formats
• Trans Fat Labeling
• Miscellaneous
• Serving Size
• Exemptions/Special Labeling Provisions

Claims
• Nutrient Content Claims
• Health Claims
• Qualified Health Claims
• Structure/Function Claims

The FDA further defines terms such as "Free," "Low," "Reduced/ Less," and "Comments" for nutrient content claims and qualified health claims for edible foods, dietary supplements for folic acid, B vitamins, selenium and cancer, antioxidant vitamins, nuts, cognitive dysfunction, dementia, heart disease, Omega-3 fatty acids, monounsaturated fatty acids, green tea, chromium picolinate, calcium, tomatoes, unsaturated fatty acids, corn oils, selenium, antioxidant vitamins, whey-protein, calculating the percent daily values for appropriate nutrients, and daily values for infants, children less than 4 years old, pregnant and lactating women.

Name and Address
• Manufacturer, packer or distributor
• Street Address
• City or town
• State
• Zip code

FoodSafety.gov is a combined FDA and the US Department of Agriculture website that lists all types of recent recalls and is a good source of recall information related to all human and animal products, including undeclared label ingredients, allergy alerts, misbranding, contaminants, and lack of import or other required inspections. Recalls due to label problems tend to dominate this list indicating strong oversight performance on the part of regulators with regard to labels [19].

The FDA also provides information on recalls and outbreaks that allow consumers and others to report problems, outbreaks, emergencies, and safety alerts.

The European Commission provides a Rapid Alert System for Food and Feed (RASFF) Portal that can be accessed for "alerts" reported by participating European countries. The presence of undeclared materials, excessive content levels, adulterants, and other label related issues are reported for European and imported products [20].

In China, the General Administration of Quality Supervision, Inspection and Quarantine of the People's Republic of China promotes their recall system to inform jittery Chinese consumers worried about food safety and quality. The Chinese system requires a Quality Supervision (QS) label for all local and imported products based on governmental standards [21].

3.2 BLENDS: WALKING ON THE EDGE

While most countries have some type of labeling law, there are many industry practices that tend to fool consumers into thinking they are receiving one product instead of another. With regards to "blends," unless a particular country, state, or region clearly specifies such things as type size, consumers may be fooled into thinking they receive one product when they are really receiving a blend. "Kona" coffee sold and distributed in the State of Hawaii (US) is a good example. Honolulu retail outlets and the Honolulu airport, in particular, have several vendors prominently displaying Kona coffee. For the unwary traveler who has heard of Kona coffee and desires to take some home as a present, it is advisable to carefully inspect the label and look for the word "blended." Lower cost packages of "Kona" coffee are lower cost for a reason. They are blended coffees containing no more than 90% coffee from some other region of the world. The minimum content of Kona coffee in these packages is 10%. The other 90% consisting of cheaper imported beans. Unwary travelers are frequently fooled by Kona Blend labels such as those shown in Figure 3.2.

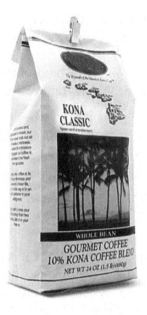
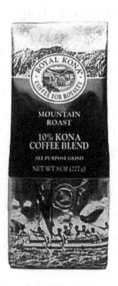

Figure 3.2 Blended Kona Coffees.

3.3 LABEL SELL BY, BEST USED BY, EXPIRATION, AND USE BY DATES

3.3.1 Packaging Controls: Sanitation and Construction

Unfortunately not all potential food fraud issues involve the simple substitution of one ingredient of a lower cost for one more expensive. Knowingly using dirty or hazardous packaging that is in contact with food products for cost savings purposes is an example of an issue not commonly recognized in conjunction with fraudulent practices. The potential for and likelihood that the packaging will adulterate the food product is often overlooked.

Preventive packaging practices are required and this means spending money early in the process. When packaging is not appropriately qualified, certified, and controlled due to cost cutting measures, adulteration becomes an issue.

The following example shows product harvest through delivery. While apple harvest and packing as used in this example are obviously not designed to intentionally or otherwise mislead consumers, the example is used to show how a packing operation can incidentally contaminate product. More importantly, the lack of controls over the packing operation sanitation can be considered a result of "economically motivated adulteration" since product is highly likely to become adulterated as a result of refusal to provide sanitary protection for the packing materials and the packing operation.

Figure 3.3 illustrates a normal apple harvest operation that is often followed by wash (Figure 3.4).

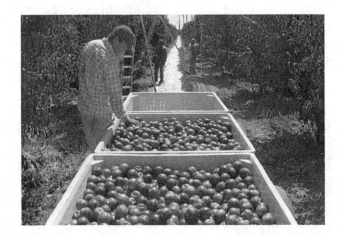

Figure 3.3 Apple Harvest.

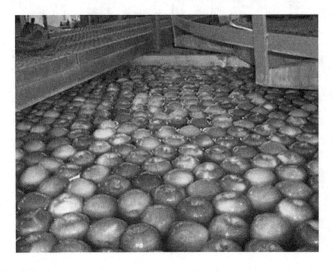

Figure 3.4 Wash Operation.

Once food is cleaned, processed, and ready for transport, the packaging that carries the food through the supply chain should be controlled to eliminate harmful outgassing, sanitized, and should protect the food from adulteration. Clean food should be moved in safe and sanitary packaging. However, money can be saved through the use of substandard and contaminated packaging. Food packaging is often mishandled in terms of appropriate sanitary control in order to save labor, space, and money.

Poor package handling and storage practices are common in the food industry. Figure 3.5 illustrates apple packs sitting in an open environment on the floor. The apples will be in contact with the inner surfaces of the cases. Other cases can be seen stacked in the

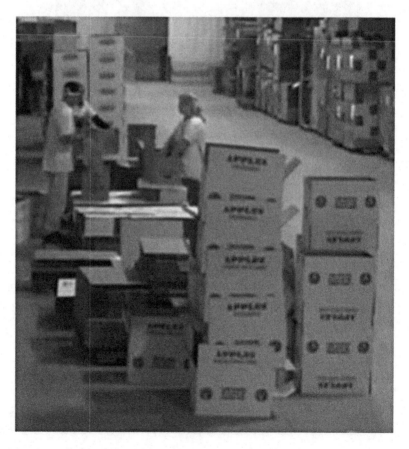

Figure 3.5 Open Environment Pack Storage and Handling.

open environment without any attempt to keep them free of contaminants. Such practices are common in the produce and fruit industries.

In July 2014, Food Safety News summarized a study published by the Food Packaging Forum that reported 175 hazardous chemicals being used in food contact packaging. The study compared lists of known hazardous packaging chemicals with lists of packaging materials used in food packaging. Food packaging is an industry that requires careful controls when the packaging ends up in contact with food. Safe and sanitary packaging is expensive to develop and control but many companies skip needed control steps. Choosing packaging that is of a lower cost when packaging may exude harmful chemicals can bring with it serious adulteration and health consequences. This is especially true when packaging is exposed to severe environments such as freezing and microwave ovens. Many of the chemicals used in food packaging are toxic and because of this, are not used in the electronics or other industries due to their abilities to destroy electronic components [22].

The original report compared European Union (EU) lists of harmful chemicals with lists of chemicals used in food packaging. The authors found that chemicals in the packaging were highly toxic. Such toxicity would not be allowed in many other products due to the ability of the chemicals to contaminate and even erode components. The electronics industry has over the past 30 years suffered significant losses due to chemical and contaminant migration and, as a result, has implemented process testing and controls. The disk drive industry commonly employs full laboratory capabilities in manufacturing plants in order to perform tests, analysis, and maintain adequate controls [23].

Food packaging requires that packaging suppliers are chosen with care, qualified, and certified by food processing operations. Some of the basic requirements for the selection of competent food packaging companies are listed in Table 3.1.

The American Society for Testing and Materials (ASTM) has published a series of standards to help identify and control package characteristics such as chemical content, acidity or alkalinity, tensile breaking strength, peel adhesion, and water, oil and tear resistance [24].

Table 3.1 Choosing the Packaging Supplier

1. Strong regulatory expertise and strict compliance protocols (certification)
2. Well defined procedures and work instructions
3. Strong product safety
4. Informed and thorough materials evaluation process (incoming and outgoing test)
5. Facility design, layout, staff, zones
6. Smart packaging design
7. Good manufacturing practices (cGMP)
8. Sanitary manufacturing practices
9. Excellent quality control staff and system
10. Rigorous material and packaging testing protocols
11. Strict handling and user requirements

ASTM test standards cover such issues as "Standard Test Method for Quantitating Non-UV-Absorbing Nonvolatile Extractables from Microwave Susceptors Utilizing Solvents as Food Simulants," "Standard Test Method for Qualitative Analysis of Volatile Extractables in Microwave Susceptors Used to Heat Food Products," and "Standard Test Method for Determining Residual Solvents in Packaging Materials." All three test standards are designed to help companies assure that chemical migration and extraction are controlled in food packaging.

The ASTM paper and packaging standards help papermaking plants, packaging and shipping companies, and other producers and end-users of paper materials and products to assure they have the proper processing and assessment procedures to ensure quality and efficient packaging suitable for commercial use.

However, the cost of such testing frequently provides a deterrent to package assurance in many food companies.

While there are many examples, the FDA weighs in on package standards through 21 CFR 175.105 covering the use of package adhesives below 120 °F; 21 CFR 177.1396 covers laminate structures over 120 °F; and 21 CFR 177.1390 covers laminate structures used over 250 °F. Failure to comply with such standards due to cost constraints or business decisions forms the basis for economically motivated adulteration of food stuffs.

Incoming packaging needs to be protected in clean zones. Assuming packaging comes into the operation in a clean and sanitary state, the packaging needs to be moved into the packing area through pass-through areas that prevent dirt from entering the packing zone. Packaging then needs to be stored in a manner that prevents contamination. In other words, the packaging itself needs to be protected from adulterants in a manner identical to the protection provided for the food and ingredients.

The state of Illinois in Sec. 1 of the (410 ILCS 650) Sanitary Food Preparation Act provides some guidance:

> *Sec. 1 That every building, room, basement, enclosure or premises, occupied, used or maintained as a bakery, confectionery, cannery, packing house, slaughter house, creamery, cheese factory, restaurant, hotel, grocery, meat market, or as a factory, shop, warehouse, any public or place or manufacturing establishment used for the preparation, manufacture, packing, storage, sale or distribution of any food as defined by statute, which is intended for sale, shall be properly and adequately lighted, drained, plumbed and ventilated, and shall be conducted with strict regard to the influence of such conditions upon the health of the operatives, employees, clerks, or other persons therein employed, and the purity and wholesomeness of the food therein produced, prepared, manufactured, packed, stored, sold or distributed.*
>
> *April 1, 2015 http://www.ilga.gov/legislation/ilcs/ilcs3.asp?*
> *ActID=1584&ChapterID=35*

Such guidance requires process controls over the package storage and packing operations. The following process control variables are considered the minimum for adequate controls:

- Temperatures
- Pressures
- Speeds
- Injection of product/gasses
- Air cleanliness controls
- Measurement
- Calibration
- Clean ability
- Sanitation

One of the most common variables frequently ignored by management is air cleanliness. Although not currently controlled in most food processing or packing operations, air cleanliness controls are certainly on the horizon as food safety and food quality controls continue to

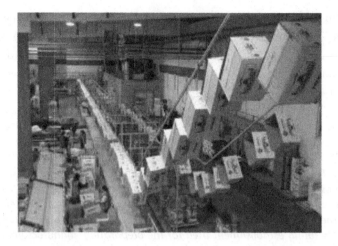

Figure 3.6 High Volume Packing.

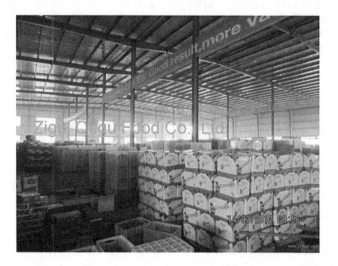

Figure 3.7 Uncontrolled Open Air Packing.

improve. While some packing lines are established for high volume packing (Figure 3.6), it can be seen that conditions conducive to maintaining clean packages are not maintained as they are open air and allow dirt from the local farm, fork lifts, and other carriers to enter the packing areas (Figures 3.7 and 3.8).

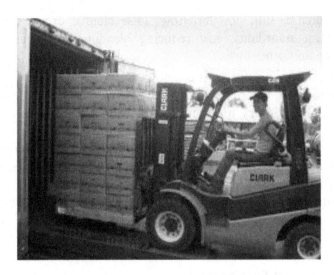

Figure 3.8 Moving Contaminants from the Packing Area to Truck Trailers.

3.4 SUPPLY CHAIN FOOD FRAUD EXAMPLES

The number of food choices a consumer may have depends greatly on suppliers, seasons, and origin locations. It is not known how widespread food fraud is throughout the world. Those who commit food fraud do so intentionally and they want to avoid detection and prosecution. However, the vast majority of food fraud incidents do not pose a public health risk. There seems to be no product that is excluded from being potentially fraudulently produced, labeled, or otherwise manipulated.

Honey
Olive Oil
Coffee
Juices
Fish
Alcohol
Dairy Products
Vitamins
Meats and Poultry

The list represents only a few of products that can be fraudulently impacted through ingredient substitution, ice and water dilution or weight increase, salt, counterfeiting, false claims, drugs, misleading labels, flame retardants, cost reducing blending, improper or dirty packaging, and other means.

3.4.1 Melamine

In 2008, diluted dairy products from China were found to include melamine used as a substitute for milk. As the demand for milk outstripped the supply, product was watered down with melamine as a way to increase the product and enhance profits. Melamine, with its high nitrogen content was added to the watered down milk to artificially inflate the protein content. 290,000 infant illnesses, 860 hospitalizations, 6 known deaths, and a $3 billion loss to industry resulted.

3.4.2 Horsemeat Sold as Beef

Ikea meatballs, Burger King hamburger patties, Cottage pies, and Frozen Lasagna were a few of the products impacted by the 2013 European horsemeat scandal. In the United Kingdom where horses are viewed as pets, people were somewhat horrified to find that they had been fooled into thinking that horsemeat was ground beef. In some countries, horsemeat is a normal product. It has the same amount of protein as beef, less fat, and poses no threat to human health (Figure 3.9).

Reportedly a breach of EU traceability regulations, forged invoices, missing records, and other irregularities all contributed to a proposal for a Food Crime Unit (FCU) and investigations indicate that implementation of EU import requirements are not being properly implemented.

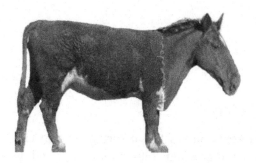

Figure 3.9 Horse Beef.

Spinoff from the horsemeat scandal continues with the jailing of some of the guilty and delays in the publication of a report seemingly embarrassing to some of the governments involved.

3.4.3 Stabilizers, Emulsions, Hydrocolloids, Flavor Enhancers, and Pink Slime

As the demand for easy to prepare processed foods grows, the demand for food stabilizers also grows. Stabilizers are basically ingredients added to food to preserve or change the food structure. Some are used to prevent component separation; others prevent the formation of ice crystals.

McDonalds has reportedly ceased the fine grinding of "trimmings" or left over meats with ammonium hydroxide added. The resulting product is now known as "pink slime." Ammonium hydroxide is added to reduce bacteria in the product which is then added to normal burger in order to increase weight and moisture content. Pink slime is approved by the United States Department of Agriculture (USDA) if used in percentages less than 25%.

As food fraud issues continue to become exposed, more and more research is being conducted to determine the extent to which the public is exposed to food fraud. In the UK, The Guardian reported in February of 2014 that testing of meat products showed that they were found to contain what is referred to as meat emulsion (or pink slime in the United States). Also many other misleading, unlabeled, or mysterious additives and substitutes had been discovered through testing of over 900 products. Over one-third of the products tested failed label comparison and ingredient tests [7].

3.4.4 Food Label Expiration Issues

Labeling is an issue that gets many companies in trouble, either accidentally or due to intentional ingredient omissions. Issues such as undeclared ingredients (milk, egg, sulfites, wheat, diclofenac, gluten, soy, peanut, and salt) may impact human health for those with allergies. In April through June 2015, the FDA listed 43 recalled food products that included everything from cumin to fresh pasta salad [25].

Twenty of the 43 recalled products (46.5%) were label issues focused on undeclared ingredients. Label issues, whether they included intentionally fraudulent omissions or not, are obviously a significant problem, especially for consumers.

Significant opportunities arise for in-market packaging professionals to commit food fraud. Placing a new date label over an "expired" food label with the intention to make the product appear to be within acceptable shelf life standards is an example. Products may also be completely repackaged and relabeled in order to avoid expired shelf life detection.

3.4.5 Label "Use By," "Best Used By," "Better if Used By," "Best if Used By," "Use Or Freeze By," "Do Not Use After," "Expiration," and other Date Labels

Is the unstandardized use of such "Use By" labels intended to inform or confuse the consumer regarding shelf life and freshness? Are such labels even defined in a general sense by food processors? While such labeling practices are commonly considered a food safety issue, the opportunity for food fraud arises among those who would substitute or promote aging contents for economic gains. The means by which a consumer or retailer could check on the validity of the label dates is missing. The issue has not been recognized as one that provides a potential for food fraud.

3.4.6 Modified Atmosphere Packaging (MAP)

Other common questionable practices include the use of carbon monoxide in meat packaging operations (usually within the store butcher's area). While in the United States the FDA considers the use of carbon monoxide generally regarded as safe (GRAS), the intent of its use is to cause the meat to appear redder than it would normally appear for extended periods of time. The FDA does not require the market using carbon monoxide to display the ingredient on labels.

The process of packaging meats, fish, and other products using modified atmosphere packaging (MAP) that use carbon monoxide is not new. When meat is placed in a Styrofoam tray in order to seal the meat and tray in plastic wrap, the tray and meat go through a packing machine that creates a carbon monoxide atmosphere during the sealing operation. The result is that the carbon monoxide is sealed in the tray with the meat. By the way, the studies that convinced the FDA to regard the process as GRAS were all conducted by the manufacturers of packaging equipment.

While the use of carbon monoxide is not considered fraudulent, consumer groups question its use without appropriate labeling.

In Europe, the European Commission under the Health and Consumer Protection Directorate-General scientific committee was asked to form an opinion "on the use of carbon monoxide as a component of packaging gasses in modified atmosphere packaging for fresh meat." Their report, adopted December 13, 2001, concludes [26]:

> The Committee therefore concluded that there is no health concern associated with the use of 0.3%–0.5% CO in a gas mixture with CO_2 and N_2 as a modified atmosphere packaging gas for fresh meat provided the temperature during storage and transport does not exceed 4 °C. However the Committee wishes to point out that, should products be stored under inappropriate conditions, the presence of CO may mask visual evidence of spoilage.

The last sentence in their concluding statement, "However the Committee wishes to point out that, should products be stored under inappropriate conditions, the presence of CO may mask visual evidence of spoilage," highlights a fraud issue for which opportunities arise in conjunction with the expiration issues noted above. Put simply, the use of carbon monoxide in meat packaging opens the door for fraudulent labeling with regard to product expiration or "best used by" dates.

Figure 3.10 depicts a CO enabled packing station and Figure 3.11 is an example of packaged beef steaks brightened by CO.

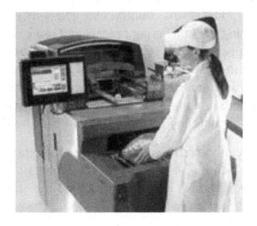

Figure 3.10 CO Packaging.

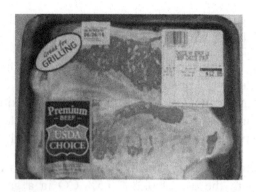

Figure 3.11 CO Packaged Steaks.

While it should be noted that the EU prohibits food companies from using carbon monoxide, US consumer groups and competitors are similarly involved in the fray. As an example, in 2005, Food Production Daily reported that a food and spice company (Kalsec) petitioned the FDA to eliminate the use of MAP in the packaging of meats. Kalsec poked the FDA for not conducting its own testing for the MAP process [27].

Carbon monoxide is also used to package fish and other products that you might see in the glass refrigerated cases in the supermarket butcher's section. For some reason, some supermarkets will place an ingredient notice in the display case revealing the fact that carbon monoxide is used in packaging while other supermarkets do not display such notices.

Consider the use of carbon monoxide to enable prepackaging of meats prior to shipping across country. One company may reduce labor costs by centralizing the butchering process and using carbon monoxide to provide the appearance of freshness. Local butchers are eliminated and the newly central location provides economies of scale. Large companies implementing such practices are in constant battles with meat cutter and butcher's unions on one hand while lobbyists continue to convince legislators that the use of carbon monoxide is GRAS.

Using carbon monoxide to preserve the appearance of freshness brings labeling, politics, laws, unions, consumers, health, and the potential for fraud into an ever twisting and unresolvable pit. Appearance has taken precedence over food safety.

3.4.7 Weight Fraud

While food expiration and appearance issues offer significant opportunities for food fraud, other simpler and more immediately useful means are available to fraudsters.

When meat or chicken or fish may be packaged in plastic, Styrofoam or other tray types and sealed with plastic, the packaging operation often involves the input of a small pad used to absorb product juices. Unfortunately, the pad can be premoistened to increase package weight.

Other types involving weight fraud are common in the fish industry where ice is added to products to skew weights. In other instances, take-out food can be a problem in fast food outlets when water is added to product. Chicken nugget products delivered through the take-out window can be easily increased in weight through the addition of water, sometimes increasing the delivered portion weight by as much as 30%. Such practices may be legal as long as water is included in the ingredient list but the ingredient list is not included with the take-out order. Figure 3.12 shows the water soaked pad that can be used to add weight to the product.

3.4.8 Not COOL

Many countries require country of origin labeling, commonly referred to as "COOL" in the United States. The intent of COOL legislation is

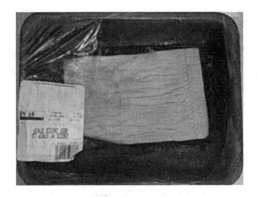

Figure 3.12 Padded Package.

to inform the consumer where the product came from as well as to control imports/exports and associated tariffs.

Mislabeling product can be advantageous to importers and exporters. Competition with "locally grown" product can be fierce and inspires some entrepreneurs to develop strategies to sell cheaper imported product under the "locally grown" or "USA" marketing umbrella. Other deceptive practices are associated with placing "local produce" signs over or near imported product in an effort to confuse the consumer as to which is locally grown and which is imported.

3.4.9 Organic Produce

Organically grown products are frequently advertised as such, and at a price higher than nonorganic produce. To the consumer, there is no way to visually determine whether or not the product was organically grown and to what organic standards. Some organic farmers are very strict with regards to seeds, soil, water and pesticide testing, and other controls commonly imposed for organic certification. Organic farming and the use of "organically grown" terminology unfortunately opens the door to all types of fraudulent practices.

It is well known that due to the sales price difference between organically grown product and nonorganically grown product some "locally grown" farmer's market entrepreneurs will secure nonorganic product at a lower price, move it to the farmer's market, and sell it at organic prices.

3.4.10 Bottled Water: Creation of Fear and Confusion

Consumers continue to increase their purchases of bottled waters out of the fear that tap water is contaminated. Generally speaking, bottled water is considered to be purer or less adulterated than tap water. But issues regarding the source and purity of the bottled water are increasing, sometimes with an overlap into questions of fraudulent labeling. For many, bottled water is considered to be the biggest food fraud scheme in history that dupes consumers out of tens of billions of dollars on an annual basis. Regardless of the true source of the water or what the label says, most households rely greatly on bottled water.

There are several types of bottled water currently marketed:

- Spring water collected by drilling into underground spring sources
- Purified water produced by distillation, reverse osmosis or other processes
- Mineral water that contains more than 250 parts per million of dissolved solids
- Sparkling bottled water that contains the same amount of carbon dioxide as it had in the source
- Artesian water or Artesian well water from a confined aquifer
- Well water from holes in the ground.

Bottled water is more highly regulated than tap water but is still mostly self-regulated. In some cases, companies treat and resell municipal tap water without disclosing the water source on the label and often under descriptors such as Ice Mountain, Desert Quench, Utopia, and Crystal Springs.

In one case, PepsiCo Inc. has agreed to add the words "public water source" to their Aquafina water labels.

Pepsi's Aquafina, and Coca-Cola Co.'s Dasani bottled waters, are both made of purified water from public reservoirs. Coca-Cola will post online consumer information about the quality control testing that goes into their bottled water, sometime near the end of summer, or early fall 2007 [28].

While the EPA regulates quality of public water supplies, bottled water is considered to be a food product and, therefore, the FDA regulates bottled water

FDA has established specific regulations for bottled water in Title 21 of the Code of Federal Regulations (21 CFR), including standard of identity regulations (21 CFR § 165.110[a]) that define different types of bottled water, such as spring water and mineral water, and standard of quality regulations (21 CFR §165.110[b]) that establish allowable levels for contaminants (chemical, physical, microbial and radiological) in bottled water. FDA also has established Current Good Manufacturing Practice (CGMP) regulations for the processing and bottling of bottled drinking water (21 CFR part 129). Labeling regulations (21 CFR part 101) and CGMP regulations (21 CFR part 110) for foods in general also apply to bottled water. It is worth noting that bottled water is one of the few foods for which FDA has developed specific CGMP regulations or such a detailed standard of quality [29].

Table 3.2 FDA Food Labeling Requirements [30]
TITLE 21—FOOD AND DRUGS
CHAPTER I—FOOD AND DRUG ADMINISTRATION DEPARTMENT OF HEALTH AND HUMAN SERVICES
SUBCHAPTER B—FOOD FOR HUMAN CONSUMPTION
PART 101—FOOD LABELING
Subpart A—General Provisions
Sec. 101.18 Misbranding of food.
(a) Among representations in the labeling of a food which render such food misbranded is a false or misleading representation with respect to another food or a drug, device, or cosmetic.
(b) The labeling of a food which contains two or more ingredients may be misleading by reason (among other reasons) of the designation of such food in such labeling by a name which includes or suggests the name of one or more but not all such ingredients, even though the names of all such ingredients are stated elsewhere in the labeling.
(c) Among representations in the labeling of a food which render such food misbranded is any representation that expresses or implies a geographical origin of the food or any ingredient of the food except when such representation is either:
(1) A truthful representation of geographical origin.
(2) A trademark or trade name provided that as applied to the article in question its use is not deceptively misdescriptive. A trademark or trade name composed in whole or in part of geographical words shall not be considered deceptively misdescriptive if it:
(i) Has been so long and exclusively used by a manufacturer or distributor that it is generally understood by the consumer to mean the product of a particular manufacturer or distributor; or
(ii) Is so arbitrary or fanciful that it is not generally understood by the consumer to suggest geographic origin.
(3) A part of the name required by applicable Federal law or regulation.
(4) A name whose market significance is generally understood by the consumer to connote a particular class, kind, type, or style of food rather than to indicate geographical origin.

Under 21 CFR part 101, the FDA calls out Food Labeling requirements as related to Misbranding of food (Table 3.2).

Five percent of the bottled water purchased in Cleveland fell within the required fluoride range recommended by the state, compared with 100% of the tap water samples, all of which were also within 0.04 mg/L of the optimal fluoride level of 1.00 mg/L. Use of bottled water based on the assumption of purity can be misguided. Recently, the Environmental Protection Agency, Washington, DC, published a final ruling that requires community water systems to regularly report to the public on the quality of local tap water; there are no similar proposals to determine the quality of bottled water through labeling [31].

3.4.11 Vitamins and Herbal Supplements

There are an estimated 65,000 dietary supplements consumed by an estimated 150 million Americans.

In February, 2015 the New York attorney general filed charges against GNC, Target, Walgreens, and Walmart when investigations found that tested products contained no herbs as indicated by their labels. Instead of herbs, fillers were found as well as some dangerous substances. The action clearly put the large retailers in the spotlight and, under rules of vicarious liability, established retailers as responsible for the food products they purchase from suppliers and sell to the public. The FDA requires companies to verify the ingredient and labeling accuracy for products the produce and sell [32].

The New York investigation was prompted by a report in the New York Timeslate in 2013 that exposed the use of fingerprinting test techniques as a means of uncovering adulteration and labeling fraud. The New York Times referenced a published research article from BMC Medicine [33].

In response, members of the herbal supplements industry have challenged the findings claiming that the testing strategies used were inadequate.

Meanwhile, during August, 2015 ConsumerLab.com continued to report on recalls and warnings for vitamins and health supplements. The list published over 800 warnings and recalls since 2002 for such issues as:

1. FDA Warns Public About Chinese Diet Pills Containing Fenfluramine
2. Maker of Eye Health Supplements Warned for Drug Claims
3. Maker of Noni, Nopal, Blood Sugar and Cholesterol Supplements Warned For Drug Claims, Misbranding, and Manufacturing Violations
4. Recall of Dalyvite Liquid Multivitamin
5. FDA Warns Company Selling Mineral Supplements as Treatments
6. Alistrol Health Inc. Warned Over Health Claims on Products
7. FDA Warns of Aloe Drug Claims and Misbranding
8. Canadian Warning on Use of Seven Herbal Supplements from BotanicLab
9. FDA Warns of Medical Claims Made For Numerous Chinese Herbal Products
10. Herbal Supplement Company Warned For Medical Claims

11. Centrum Multivitamins: Breast and Colon Health Claims Pulled
12. Maker of Pain Relief, Virility, and Idebenone Products Warned of Violations by FDA [34].

3.4.12 Food is Cash: Theft and Resale

Not all steps in the supply chain illustration above lend themselves to some of the food fraud definitions noted. Substitution of products at distributor, packing, chiller, palletizing, and shelf points allow for some products to be substituted for others while truck transportation offer opportunities for food theft. Food is the number one product stolen during transportation and resold during through fenced markets. With over $30 billion of cargo stolen annually, food and drink represent the hottest targets. Generally food shipment thefts are by "deceptive pickup" (thieves posing as drivers receive loads from unwary shippers) or from unsecured parking [35].

The average loss per incident exceeds $600,000 and costs shippers and carriers $30-$50 million each year. The black market for food heats up during bad economic times and includes just about every type of food you can imagine. Stolen food typically fetches 70 cents on the dollar compared to 30 cents or less for electronics, the second most popular target for thieves.

Cheese, eggs, milk, beer, nonalcoholic beverages, produce, and just about any food product can become hijacker targets. The fact that food products may provide a risk/reward return for thieves means that many of them can end up in many retail markets whose managers are working to increase profit margins. Stolen food purchased at 70 cents on the dollar means the retailer has added significantly to net profits.

Food theft is accomplished through a variety of ways. Sometimes the driver is involved. On other occasions, well organized gangs are active in deceptively picking up loads and trailers or stealing the trailer or food container in its entirety. With the top food theft states including California, Florida, Texas, and New Jersey, stolen food becomes fraudulent food that will see later sales to unscrupulous retailers. Food is stolen from warehouses, distribution centers, parking lots, truck stops, and other unsecured locations with Fridays and Saturdays being the favorite days to conduct the theft.

When food is stolen, the FDA is "committed to work with the affected firm to minimize the public health risks and ensure an appropriate public health response" and "has developed streamlined procedures to rapidly respond to reports of theft and ensure consistency as we work with firms that have experienced a cargo or warehouse theft [36]."

3.4.13 Transshipment Fraud

Transshipment is a means of fraud that includes the transfer of a shipment from one carrier or vessel to another during transit, usually to hide the identity of the port or country of origin. The act of laundering honey represents one of the largest food fraud cases in the United States' history. Honey is one of the top ten products involved in food fraud in the world.

In 2006, the US Department of Homeland Security and the US Department of Commerce uncovered a plot by a German company named the ALW Food Group to import honey into the United States by buying honey in China and shipping it in 55 gallon drums to other ports. The other ports included India, Malaysia, South Korea, Russia, Mongolia, Thailand, Taiwan, and the Philippines. At each new port, the honey was relabeled to show it was from those ports and US import documents were falsified. Due to increased US import fees on Chinese honey, ALW was looking for ways to fraudulently import the honey to their US customers without paying the increased fees.

A number of company executives were indicted on global conspiracy charges as a result of their involvement in this $80 million dollar scam [37].

CHAPTER 4

Unprotected Customers

4.1 DETECTION TESTING AND THE AUTHENTICATION DILEMMA

The choice of analytical test development and methods are primarily determined by preexisting knowledge of the potential adulterant. That means that until an illegal substitute causes a problem, no one tests for the substituted ingredient. Further, perhaps there is no known test for the substitute. There is simply no way of knowing who could put what into what in order to save money or change the appearance of a product. In short, the food industry is constantly lagging in detection test technology. Testing for ingredient substitutes is not a preventive strategy.

The US Pharmacopeial (USP) the Food Fraud Database offers users the ability to search for food fraud cases and to report food fraud cases [38].

The search function allows a user to enter a term such as "peanut" which provides a list of relatively recent filings. By clicking on the "+" symbol, a user can look at the "Reported Detection Method" and reference information.

A search on the word peanut, for example, provides the type of testing used to determine whether or not peanut products (oil, flavor, etc.) were used in the product. Fatty acid fingerprinting, GC-FID for FAME analysis, DNA analysis by PCR-CE-single-strand conformation polymorphism, and low field NMR to measure transverse relaxation distributions were returned by the USP system in a recent search.

A similar search for fraudulent honey testing returns amino acid fingerprinting by gas chromatography (GC), amino acids and proteins fingerprinting by high performance liquid chromatography (HPLC), protein fingerprinting by SDS-PAGE, physiochemical properties with chemometrics, pollen analysis, saccharides profile by GC-MS, saccharides profile by HPLC, and others. Much of the reporting in the USP database

Food Fraud. DOI: http://dx.doi.org/10.1016/B978-0-12-803393-7.00004-4

is characterized as "scholarly," related to "Honey of nonauthentic geographic or botanical origin" and "replacement" food fraud incidents. Many of the scholarly articles are summaries of research conducted to determine faster, more accurate, and less expensive substitute food fraud testing. For example, Arvanitoyannis et al. in Food Science and Nutrition (January 12, 2007) in an article entitled "Novel Quality Control Methods in Conjunction with Chemometrics (Multivariate Analysis) for Detecting Honey Authenticity" summarize their research with the following:

> The importance of honey has been recently upgraded because of its nutrient and therapeutic effect. The adulteration of honey increased exponentially in terms of both geographic and/or botanical origin. Therefore, the need has arisen for more effective quality control methods aiming at detecting adulteration. Various novel, fast, and accurate methods like AAS, HPLC, GC-MS, ES-MS, TLC, HPAED-PAD, NMR, FT-Raman, and NIR have enriched the arsenal of analytical chemist in this direction. However, apart from these novel methods, the application of multivariate analysis and, in particular, PCA, CLA, and CA, proved to be extremely useful for grouping and detecting honey of various origins. Mineral and trace element analysis were repeatedly shown to be a very effective means for the classification purposes of honey of various origins (geographical and botanical) [39].

http://www.tandfonline.com/doi/abs/10.1080/10408690590956369?
journalCode=bfsn20

As authentication testing continues to evolve, undoubtedly those adopting test strategies and purchasing equipment for particular adulterant situations will continue their search for low cost, rapid, accurate approaches that suit their testing needs. Considering the previous few paragraphs that illustrate the variety of testing approaches for single adulterants, finding the best test will not be an easy task. Those in need of test solutions have a couple of options open: Set up a lab and conduct in-house testing, or send samples to labs. Setting up a lab requires high capital costs not conducive to small companies while sending samples to labs means ongoing expenses.

With food recalls in the daily news, consumers are understandably becoming more and more jittery to the point where many may be seen in the supermarket using their cell phone bar code readers to read labels. Many labels include within the bar code information related to the producer or processor. But how does reading bar code labels help boost consumer trust?

Knowing which foods are most at risk may help. In October, 2013, Forbes listed the "Top 10 'At Risk' Fraudulent Foods and Why You Should Feel Scammed." Included in the list (in order) were [40]:

1. Olive oil
2. Fish
3. Organic foods
4. Milk
5. Grains
6. Honey and maple syrup
7. Coffee and tea
8. Spices
9. Wine
10. Fruit juices

The idea that food fraud can be prevented is based on the idea that risk can be assessed and controlled. Under quality cost control conditions, testing, purity testing, or identity testing of product or ingredients is not considered a preventive strategy. Preventive approaches are proactive and involve causal analysis as a means of permanently removing causes through continuous improvement of operational processes.

While most professionals would look at an incoming test as a preventive strategy, ingredient or product testing is expensive and a burden to all members of the supply chain. However, test and inspection are frequently the first strategies victim companies afraid of food fraud are likely to turn to and install as part of their overall operational controls.

From a quality perspective, prevention costs include such things as planning, establishment of industry standards, supplier qualification and certification, and employee training and education are all approaches that require up-front effort on the part of food suppliers and receivers.

Recall of fraudulent products is considered an external failure cost and, as such, is the most expensive quality system failure. Again, many food safety professionals consider recall as a preventive strategy, but it is clearly not, it is reactive. Using the reasoning that recall prevents further damage, many will argue its preventive nature in terms of recapture and removal of fraudulent products. Recall is not proactive, nor does it require causal analysis to remove initial causes. Recall is reactive and is an attempt to recapture the horse after it has escaped from the barn. The gate needs to be locked long before the horse escapes.

As in any food safety or food quality failure, the product that has been fraudulently installed into the supply chain has usually been identified as an escape and is not the subject of what are more commonly called corrective actions (i.e., locate, recapture, disposal). Other preventive strategies may be employed including training, research, working with involved groups, attending public meetings, and joining organizations to discuss findings and issues.

While some fraud is considered not harmful to humans, the fact that fraud was intentional in order to save money brings the act of fraud into the legal arena. Once fraud is discovered, recall activities, traceability back to the source, and investigations regarding the source of the fraud begin and enforcement professionals become involved.

4.2 WHISTLE BLOWERS

Food fraud is often reported by whistle blowers. In 2013, NBC News reported that Sysco, one of the largest food distributors in the United States, was temporarily storing perishable food in dirty unrefrigerated storage sheds in the San Francisco Bay area. The information came from whistle blowers. Sysco refrigerated trucks were delivering product to different regions, placing the product into storage sheds for delivery by regional sales personnel to various restaurant and other clients. NBC investigators watched as Sysco sales personnel opened the storage sheds, retrieved some of the food (eggs, milk, seafood, raw meat, produce, etc.) and placed the product in the trunk of their cars. News personnel recorded temperatures in the sheds reaching over 80 °F. In some instances, the sales person, after loading their trunks with food, stopped for lunch prior to delivering the product [41].

Further investigation found that Sysco followed this practice in other parts of the United States and in Canada. While Sysco refused to publically discuss the issue, they issued a couple of comments. The first was this: "Effective immediately, all products delivered by Sysco San Francisco will be transported by Sysco-owned vehicles." The second comment issued was to the effect that personnel responsible for this delivery strategy were terminated which was followed by "In addition to the settlement with the state, we have comprehensively addressed our food safety and quality assurance practices in California and across the Sysco enterprise."

NBC News later reported that Sysco was fined $19.4 million by the California Department of Public Health (CDPH) and the California Food Drug and Medical Device Task Force. Company records between July 2009 and August 2013 revealed that 7 distribution centers and 25 drop sites were involved in delivering 405, 859 food items in unregistered drop sites, some of which were delivered to hospitals and schools. Of these, over 156,000 food items were considered to be potentially hazardous. Sysco conducted a voluntary recall of some of the products [42].

The CDPH investigative report is available at [43].

The report includes the following violations for various Sysco drop sites:

- It is unlawful to store food in an unregistered facility
- It is unlawful to sell, deliver, hold, or offer for sale any misbranded food
- It is unlawful to sell, deliver, hold, or offer for sale any adulterated food
- It is unlawful to hold potentially hazardous food above 45 °F.

One might assume that individuals and companies identified as the source of economically motivated food fraud are likely to have committed other acts of a fraudulent nature and investigations led to research regarding other products that have been produced and shipped.

The interesting thing about this is that Sysco cites "High-Tech Tools for Fighting Food Fraud" on its website. Included are discussions of DNA testing and isotope analysis. On the same page, they state "Advanced logistics, supply-chain management and traceability also play important roles in fighting food fraud. Our rigorous supplier approval process is designed to identify trustworthy, dependable supply sources that share our commitment to product quality and brand integrity. We also maintain thorough checks to ensure that all items are accurately measured and properly labeled."

"Sysco utilizes innovative approaches like these to ensure the quality and reliability of our products—from our suppliers to your doors."

Sysco's motto is "Good things come from Sysco" [44].

While one company may follow practices that save them money at the expense of adulteration, other companies follow practices that exude higher integrity. Maintaining quality and food safety controls over food products is a company issue. Different business practices, leadership philosophies, and day-to-day implementation, when working together, prevent companies from following fraudulent practices that might harm consumers. While the FDA requires companies to self-report food safety violations and to conduct appropriate recalls, those that do not are following fraudulent practices.

Kraft foods, as an example, found that a supplier had not stored or maintained an ingredient at required temperatures. The ingredient was used in the production of 7000 cases of American singles cheese with "best used by" dates in February, 2015. Kraft voluntarily recalled the product "as a precaution." Exactly why Kraft recalled the product is open to question but the recall itself speaks to the need for the company to follow business practices that intend to comply with laws [45].

4.3 WHAT ARE CONSUMERS BEING TOLD?

Mercola.com and others are working to develop recommendations that provide consumer food fraud guidance. Among Dr Joseph Mercola's recommendations in a 2013 article entitled "Food Fraud: What Are You Really Eating?" are the following:

- Buy the whole fish so you can recognize the species
- Buy fresh food from local producers
- Reduce dependence on processed foods
- Limit purchases of foods requiring extensive label ingredient lists
- Read the label [46].

The immature state of ingredient testing, dependence on whistle blowing and intentional violation of common food safety standards by major food supply players leave customers and consumers exposed to many types of food fraud.

CHAPTER 5

Traceability and Temperature Monitoring: Building Chain of Custody Systems

Product traceability has been determined to be of significance in terms of its ability to allow members of the supply chain, including consumers, to know where a particular product has come from, and to establish a means of recall in case the product was somehow fraudulently adulterated at one or another handling stage. Taking quick corrective action is critical to protecting the reputation of the supply chain. The move from one-up and one-down traceability to chain of custody systems is also critical to establishing legal responsibilities.

In 2009, the Institute of Food Technologists (IFT) published the first of a number of traceability reports for the FDA. The IFT has been contracted to complete and submit many more specific traceability reports since that time. The IFT has consistently emphasized the need for requiring data standardization through the past several years. The FDA has published no traceability standards. Consideration was given for traceability of food products from the harvest site (including date and time) through the retail outlet. As of this writing, the IFT has established the Global Food Traceability Center and has published a number of traceability reports for the FDA [47].

Traceability of products from the origin through the retail outlet is critical to the protection of consumers, brands and suppliers in case of fraudulent food recalls. The speed with which the source of the fraudulent food is identified and the speed with which all locations of all products shipped in the fraud lot can be identified helps to reduce impact on innocent suppliers. Once fraudulent food enters the supply chain, two types of recall may be initiated. Trade level recalls generally mean that the food has not yet left the supply chain and has not yet been sold to consumers. Consumer recalls represent the most expensive and time consuming type of recall. Consumers must be notified, generally through the mass media, to remove fraudulent products from their own food storage areas.

Food Fraud. DOI: http://dx.doi.org/10.1016/B978-0-12-803393-7.00005-6

Consumer recalls often result in consumers refusing to buy any related product because they are not sure whether or not nonimpacted products are not fraudulent. The impact of consumer recalls on the overall supply chain can result in hundreds of millions of dollars in lost sales.

While traceability solutions from technology suppliers worldwide abound, many food supply companies have moved beyond simple slap-and-ship barcode labels and have reached a level of sophistication that allows consumers to access product origin and condition information. Food traceability may be required at different levels including traceability of the individual item (item traceability), a package or carton of items (case level traceability), pallet, or container level traceability (at the truck trailer or shipping level).

5.1 ITEM LEVEL TRACEABILITY

Item level traceability refers to the application of a barcode to each package or each item in the package or shipping case. As an example, individual apples may be tracked using labels that contain information related to the supplier, product and individual apple identifier.

There is also an ongoing attempt by several companies to develop radio frequency identification (RFID) inks that are readable using RFID readers. However, at this time, the technology is not yet at a level where it is functional through the food chain. The development of RFID inks used in labels and on individual items would significantly reduce the cost of applying RFID technology in the food industry. Current RFID technology using passive tags have been used in pilot studies to track and trace at the case level, but are not suitable for item level traceability. At the case level, preprinted RFID passive tags cost over 10 cents each and are not considered to be a cost effective solution when compared to barcode solutions.

Item level traceability is more commonly applied to the packages consumers purchase in the retail outlet. Each package has a unique label applied, by either using an externally applied label or by printing the barcode directly on the package.

5.2 BARCODE: CASE LEVEL TRACEABILITY

Barcode offers supply chain members the cheapest approach to case level traceability with labels applied on automated packaging lines at a cost of fractions of a penny per label. With downloadable barcode reading apps

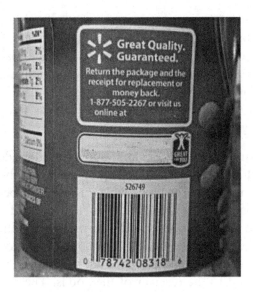

Figure 5.1 The Use of Barcodes for Item Level Traceability.

available for free for most cell phones, some information is available to shoppers. Barcode solutions are generally used at the item and case levels (Figure 5.1).

One simple solution to the implementation of a barcode system is for a distribution center to supply preprinted rolls of barcode labels to each product supplier. In this case, the distributor identifies each product coming from each supplier and supplies an adequate supply of preprinted label rolls to the supplier. The supplier then simply applies the tag to a specified position on each case prior to shipping to the distribution center. Incoming product at the distribution is often read with data going into the distribution center inventory location system. When product is shipped out of the distribution center, the barcode is read a second time to record the removal of product from inventory.

5.3 PALLET LEVEL TRACEABILITY AND TEMPERATURE MONITORING

In some instances, suppliers and shippers have good reasons to track complete pallets, often loaded with 20 or more cases of food. A simple scenario includes barcoded cases loaded on a single pallet which has its own independent tag. The pallet level tag often records the relative temperature and has its own unique identification number. When the pallet full of cases ships, all case level barcodes are read and the pallet tag (including temperature) is also read. Data for both the case bar-codes and the pallet tag are then "associated" using software technology. The assumption is that the cases on the pallet are being transported under the temperature control conditions recorded by pallet level tag. The software that "associates" the case with the pallet then provides a record for each case that includes the pallet tag temperature reading.

Shippers, carriers, receivers, and auditors often depend on this upgraded pallet level system of tracking to verify supply chain temperature controls required for perishable products. Upcoming FSMA Rules on the Sanitary Transportation of Human and Animal Foods require that the shipper specify to the carrier appropriate temperature controls with the carrier responsible for maintaining those controls and for being able to report temperature and, sometimes, GPS data back to the shipper and to the receiver of the goods. The rules also require the establishment of record systems that must be made available to food safety and governmental auditors upon demand.

From a food fraud perspective, economically motivated adulteration is often found when it is discovered that the carrier has intentionally turned off the reefer system in food transportation units. This is done in order to save fuel and has been reported on a number of occasions by the news media and a number of police departments. In August 2012, Jeff Rossen of Today worked with the Indiana State Police to watch as they stopped food carrying trucks that had intentionally turned off reefers. Other drivers continued deliveries even though they knew the refrigeration units were not working and chicken, meat, milk, and other perishable products had spoiled. Figure 5.2 shows chicken juice drooling from a frozen food package that had been defrosted during transportation. Figure 5.3 shows the Indiana State Police tossing spoiled food into the back of a dump truck for later disposal [48].

More expensive and sophisticated solutions designed to actually track and trace product through the supply chain involve several components related to product identity, real-time tracking, condition (sanitation, temperature, and humidity), history, and cost. Global Systems 1 (GS1) has designed and established a number of standards designed to allow food suppliers to identify not only the food product's origin but its product identity and a numerical identifier for the specific

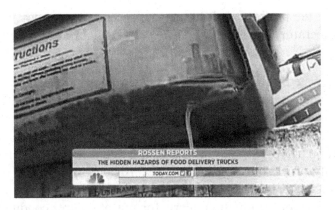

Figure 5.2 Melting Chicken.

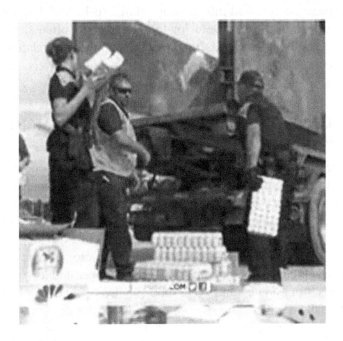

Figure 5.3 Police Unload.

package containing the product. Such systems are established to provide unique item identity and to provide traceability back to the site of origin and to enhance recall requirements in the event of adulteration. Other traceability solutions currently being developed in anticipation of the upcoming finalization of FSMA rules, represent a new generation of technology that includes cell phone, Bluetooth and other wireless technologies capable of providing information relative to the identity of the product, its location at a specific time of day, its condition (temperature, humidity), and a complete data history designed to allow for rapid recall.

These systems are known as identity, location, and condition (ILC) systems. They are generally relatively easy to install, require little or no maintenance or technical expertise, are wireless, use cell phone technology, and are useful throughout the supply chain for providing load level information. ILC systems represent the future target for enhanced traceability systems capable of not only providing one-up and one-back functions, but providing management, traceability, shelf life controls, real-time locator information, alerts for out of control conditions, and add significant other bits of data such as sanitation, security, container maintenance records, and information related to FDA FSMA sanitary food transportation rules. Data for these systems is often stored in on external computers known as the cloud making it and related reports simultaneously accessible for shippers, carriers, and receivers.

5.4 PALLET AND CONTAINER LEVEL TRACEABILITY AND TEMPERATURE MONITORING

There are a number of products available that can be used to monitor individual pallet temperatures or, when placed on the shipping container or reefer walls, are suitable for monitoring the location, time, date, and temperature within the container. One of the newest products that is reasonably priced, easy to install (requires no technical expertise, wiring, or system administration), works on Bluetooth technology, shares information via the cloud, can be remotely configured (upper and lower temperature limits for email and cell phone alerts), and is FCC and internationally certified runs at a price around $100 per unit. Bluetooth provides cell phone connectivity which means that the shipper, carrier, and receiver can all simultaneously access temperature and location data.

A free app is downloaded from the Internet that allows the user to remotely configure the unit and read location, date, time, and location data in real time. The unit comes with an option to have it calibrated (a food safety requirement) and to permanently store data collected on the pallet or container in the cloud (about $13 per year per unit). Each unit runs on a lithium battery, which is replaceable, and the unit can be attached to the pallet or container wall using the

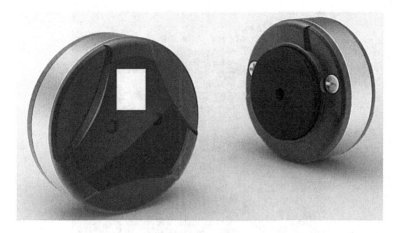

Figure 5.4 Pallet/Container Unit.

external magnet or an adhesive. The unit (Figure 5.4) is approximately two inches in diameter. The metal ring around the outside of the unit collects ambient temperature data and is sensitive to rapid temperature changes. The cell phone screen temperature display is depicted in Figure 5.5.

5.5 CONTAINER LEVEL TRACEABILITY AND TEMPERATURE CONTROL

As an example, one container level management system is designed to use cell phone, global positioning, and Wi-Fi technology to establish comprehensive data collection for shippers, carriers, receivers, and reefer or container traceability and maintenance. The system employs one or more temperature measuring tag(s) within the container. The tag passes temperature data through the cell phone to the cloud. A free downloadable application is loaded into the cell phone or tablet. Data related to the overall container shipment load, sanitation, and maintenance are entered into the application, and matched with the tag identification which is tied to the container identification number. The system (Figure 5.6) allows anyone involved with the condition of the shipment, including sanitizing, loading, unloading, or maintaining the container, to easily record data related to the particular load.

Figure 5.7 shows the cell phone or tablet temperature trends and Figure 5.8 shows the GPS location data.

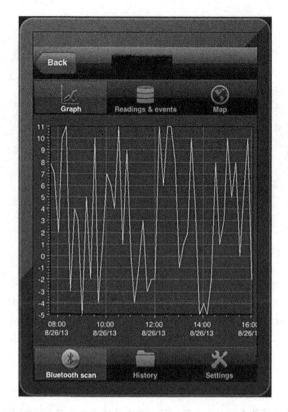

Figure 5.5 Cell Phone Temperature Display.

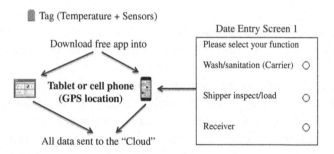

Figure 5.6 Container Traceability and Monitoring System.

Figure 5.9 shows how the user can input wash/sanitation, shipper, receiver, and maintenance data by clicking on the blue button. The "Shipper Load Data Entry Screen" shown in Figure 5.10 allows the supervisor in charge of loading the reefer or container to enter

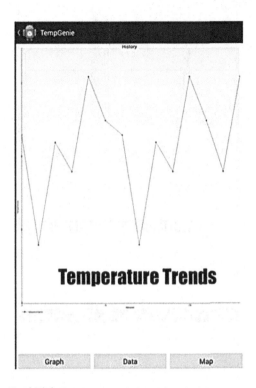

Figure 5.7 Temperature Trend Display.

significant information about the load. This information records, with single clicks, whether or not the load is refrigerated, for human or animal consumption, perishable, requires special handling, whether or not security seals are installed, and whether temperatures are recorded in degrees F or C.

Figure 5.11 allows the shipment unload operation to check security seals, sanitation inspection, and temperatures against shipper and receiver requirements. Figure 5.12 allows the container or trailer wash crew to record temperatures, chemicals, testing, inspection, and temperature data. Figure 5.13 provides anyone in the supply chain to record maintenance required for the reefer or the container itself.

By knowing the identity, condition, and location of food products in transportation at the container level in combination with pallet and case level (barcode) labels, traceability systems have come a long way

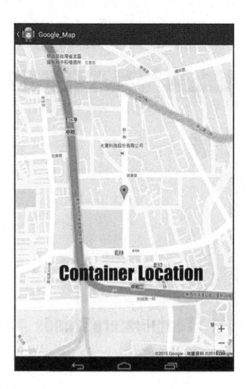

Figure 5.8 GPS Display.

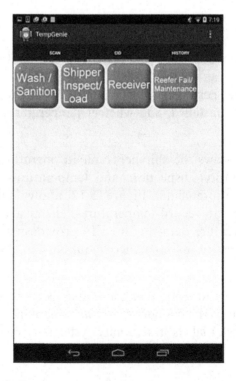

Figure 5.9 Location Selection.

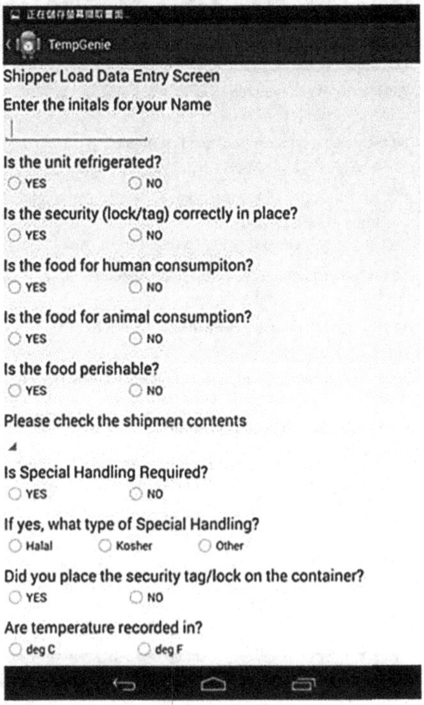

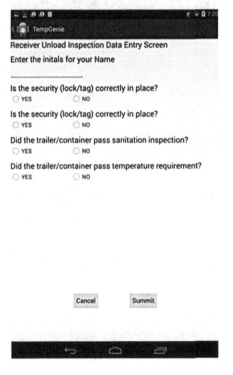

TempGenie

Shipper Load Data Entry Screen

Enter the initals for your Name

Is the unit refrigerated?
○ YES   ○ NO

Is the security (lock/tag) correctly in place?
○ YES   ○ NO

Is the food for human consumpiton?
○ YES   ○ NO

Is the food for animal consumption?
○ YES   ○ NO

Is the food perishable?
○ YES   ○ NO

Please check the shipmen contents

Is Special Handling Required?
○ YES   ○ NO

If yes, what type of Special Handling?
○ Halal   ○ Kosher   ○ Other

Did you place the security tag/lock on the container?
○ YES   ○ NO

Are temperature recorded in?
○ deg C   ○ deg F

Figure 5.10 Shipper Data Entry.

TempGenie

Receiver Unload Inspection Data Entry Screen

Enter the initals for your Name

Is the security (lock/tag) correctly in place?
○ YES   ○ NO

Is the security (lock/tag) correctly in place?
○ YES   ○ NO

Did the trailer/container pass sanitation inspection?
○ YES   ○ NO

Did the trailer/container pass temperature requirement?
○ YES   ○ NO

Cancel   Summit

Figure 5.11 Unload Data Entry.

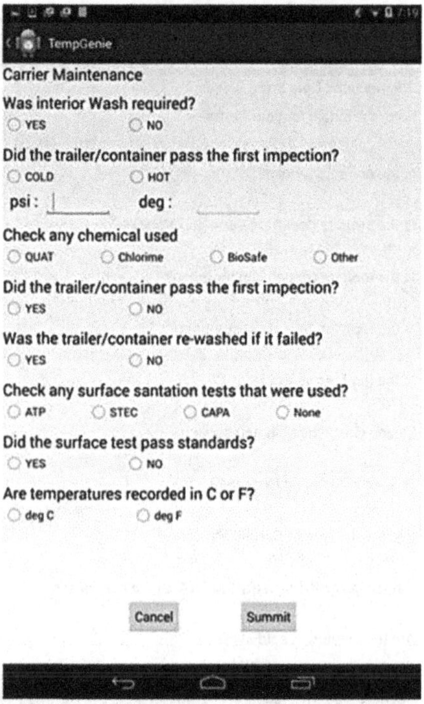

Figure 5.12 Carrier Record.

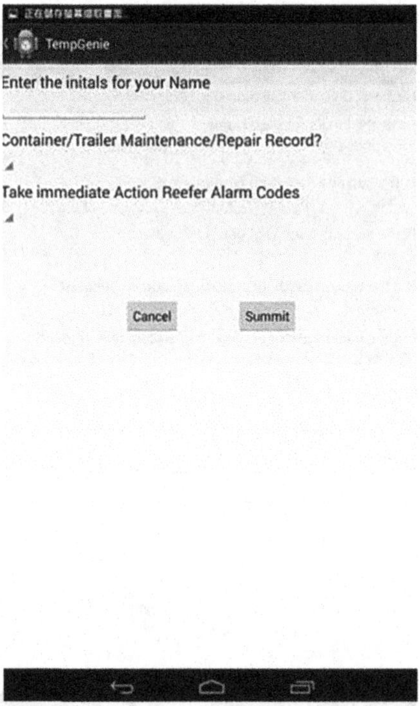

Figure 5.13 Reefer Maintenance Record.

since 2009. Records related to each shipment's condition and maintenance provide significant tracking and management information for stolen or fraudulent food loads. Such records are also critically important in terms of recalling fraudulent foods and tracking their routes through the supply chain.

The system also includes a section to allow for container and reefer maintenance. Using standard container descriptors and the Thermo King reefer alarm codes, two drop down menus allow the user to enter maintenance and problem record data relative to the container or trailer reefer. This data is entered using the Container/Reefer Maintenance Data Entry Screen which records the location of the maintenance, time/date, initials of the inspector, driver, or maintenance person, and other data.

Tables 5.1 and 5.2 provide details for the container and reefer maintenance records.

Maintaining container and reefer maintenance data provides information that allows container and reefer owners to analyze container and fleet level problems that might need attention in order to prevent fraudulently transporting foods adulterated from external sources or reefer failure. Tag and container identification numbers are standardized and individualized using RFID and GS1's (Serial Shipping Container Codes (SSCC)) coding system.

Table 5.1 Container/Trailer Maintenance Repair Record Data Entry Screen

1 Door
2 Gaskets
3 Retaining Strips
5 Chute
6 Seal
7 Floor
8 Roof
9 Wall Panel
11 Ducting
13 Rails
14 Drains
15 Cross Members
16 Insulation
17 Electrical Circuitry
18 Lock
19 Other

Table 5.2 Take immediate Action Reefer Alarm Codes Data Entry Screen	
Code	**Problem Area**
10	HIGH DISCHARGE PRESSURE (OR TEMP)
12	SENSOR OR DIGITAL INPUT SHUTDOWN
23	COOLING CYCLE FAULT
24	HEATING CYCLE FAULT
27	VAPOR MOTOR RPM HIGH (CR)
32	REFRIGERATION CAPACITY LOW
35	CHECK RUN RELAY CIRCUIT
36	ELECTRIC MOTOR FAILED TO RUN
38	ELECTRIC PHASE REVERSED
44	CHECK FUEL SYSTEM
47	REMOTE SENSOR SHUTDOWN
48	CHECK BELTS OR CLUTCH
60	CHECK BOOST CIRCUIT
62	AMMETER OUT CALIBRATION
63	ENGINE OR VAPOR MOTOR STOPPED
66	LOW ENGINE OIL LEVEL
75	CONTROLLER RAM FAILURE
76	CONTROLLER EPROM FAILURE
77	CONTROLLER EPROM CHECKSUM FAILURE
78	DATA LOG EPROM FAILURE
82	HIGH COMPRESSOR TEMP SHUTDOWN
90	ELECTRIC OVERLOAD
91	CHECK ELECTRIC READY INPUT
93	LOW COMPRESSOR SUCTION PRESSURE
97	FAILED REMOTE RETURN AIR SENSOR
99	HIGH COMPRESSOR PRESSURE RATIO
101	CONTROLLING ON EVAP COIL OUTLET TEMP
102	LOW EVAPORATOR COIL TEMPERATURE
114	MULTIPLE ALARMS-CAN NOT RUN

5.6 RECALL AND THE CHAIN OF CUSTODY

Webster's New World Law Dictionary defines chain of custody as "The order of places where, and the persons with whom, physical evidence was located from the time it was collected to its submission at trial" [49].

Wikipedia further defines chain of custody as "in legal contexts, refers to the chronological documentation or paper trail, showing the seizure, custody, control, transfer, analysis, and disposition of physical or electronic evidence.

Particularly important in criminal cases, the concept is also applied in civil litigation—and sometimes more broadly in drug testing of athletes, traceability of food products and to provide assurances that wood products originate from sustainably managed forests" [50].

With such new traceability and reporting technology presently available and others on the horizon, future capabilities for monitoring, controlling, locating, and recalling fraudulent foods are at an all-time high and bound to improve drastically over the next decade. Applying chain of custody practices for the purposes of food traceability and monitoring can have a significant impact on the prosecution of food fraud practitioners.

Real-time traceability and temperature monitoring systems are supposed to be capable of quickly identifying food origins and, more importantly, the location of all related product throughout the supply chain. Thus time-to-recall can be greatly reduced thus providing regulators and the food supply chain with the capability to greatly reduce brand damage, recall costs and human exposure. While some consider recall to be a preventive exercise through erroneous reasoning that confuses corrective action with preventive action, the recall exercise is still of critical importance. Once the fraudulent food enters the supply chain, distribution channels can take it in any of hundreds of directions through hundreds of logistical routes.

Current recall strategies frequently rely on paper "one up/one back" traceability systems that leave all supply chain members exposed for the duration of the recall. Real-time systems support rapid recall of fraudulent product thus limiting the exposure of associated brand names and work to reduce human exposure to problem foods.

When the FDA responds to or issues a recall, their approach to tracking down the problem is not complex. They use objective sampling and testing to confirm the source of the recall. What the FDA does not tell anyone is that the extent of bacterial contamination is so widespread on farms and so diverse that they have no idea how to control the causes, especially those of a bacterial nature. In 2008 during the tomato recall, the FDA held a number of 50 state conference calls during which they exposed the fact that most of the farms they sampled for contaminants were, indeed, contaminated with various types of adulterants and bacteria. While the FDA did not find the specific strain they searched for, what they did find was that many food and water samples showed contamination from fecal coliform and generic *Escherichia coli*. The information was discussed during the 50-state conference call. No public disclosures of the findings were disseminated.

Withholding such information from the general public smacks of FDA involvement in fraudulently allowing adulterant product to enter the food supply chain. It could be reasoned that the FDA and the federal, state, and local governmental officials on the phone call recognized the fact that disclosure would throw newly evolving food safety laws and implementation efforts into turmoil. More importantly, informing the public that the FDA and the professionals paid as government officials purposely withheld such information most likely would threaten not only their jobs, but any faith the public and congress might have in the FDA's ability to cope with food safety problems. Certainly, government funding for support of the FSMA and the FDA could be jeopardized. While it might not be considered to be in the public's best interest to disclose such information, a tie between economic gain and deliberate deception is established.

The situation regarding what the FDA and other agencies should do about uncontrollable levels of food contamination at the farm remains to this day. In today's world, the technology is simply not available to assure that, as an example, water sources and irrigation systems are capable of being maintained at a level where fecal coliform and bacteria are adequately controlled and eliminated to the point where adulterants do not contaminate produce.

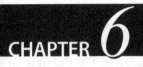

CHAPTER 6

Recommendations

Understanding that not all food fraud is intentional but may be the result of what are today considered normal business practices helps to form the basis or more preventive food fraud systems. Food fraud can, because of such normal business practices, impact any supplier-customer link throughout the supply chain and result in recalls impacting all participants. With this thinking in mind, there are several recommendations that can be made that are supportive of more preventive practices than those commonly followed today.

6.1 ESTABLISH CHAIN OF CUSTODY AS A STANDARDIZED FOOD SUPPLY CHAIN TRACEABILITY REQUIREMENT

Those individuals and companies that create illusions and practice fraud and deception in the food supply chain are, in general, intent on hiding themselves and what they do or fail to do. Causing all members of the supply chain to participate in a chain of custody traceability system should become a basic supplier requirement. Deterring fraud through requirements to participate in and use of standardized chain of custody is used in other industries to provide for product and customer protection. Fraudsters will find it much more difficult to hide. Enforcement will have the data they need to recall and prosecute. The time it takes to recall fraudulent product will be reduced. Innocent food suppliers and consumers will be protected.

6.2 TAKE RESPONSIBILITY

It should be clear that food fraud whether or not intentional, harmful, or economically motivated has many faces, most of them intentionally hidden from public view. Pretending that food fraud cannot impact any supply chain member is naïve and irresponsible.

Food Fraud. DOI: http://dx.doi.org/10.1016/B978-0-12-803393-7.00006-8

Vicarious liability is defined by Wikipedia as "a form of strict, secondary liability that arises under the common law doctrine of agency—*respondeat superior*—the responsibility of the superior for the acts of their subordinate, or, in a broader sense, the responsibility of any third party that had the 'right, ability or duty to control' the activities of a violator." Any food supply company that does not provide due diligence in the form of qualification, certification and oversight for any supplier is, indeed, somewhat responsible for the act of their suppliers.

On the international level, Codex Alimentarius (http://www.codexa-limentarius.org), goes further in calling out supply chain member consumer protection responsibilities in its Principles and Guidelines for National Food Control Systems (CAC/GL 82-2013).

52. Control programs should be applied at the point or points in the production or supply chain where hazards can be most effectively or efficiently controlled taking into account the available resources and capability. Control programs amongst other things may cover, as appropriate:

- Establishments, installations, equipment, personnel, and material;
- Products, from raw material to the final products, including intermediate products;
- Preventative controls including Good Agricultural Practice (GAP), Good Manufacturing Practices (GMP), Good Hygiene Practices (GHP), and Hazard Analysis Critical Control Point (HACCP) principles;
- Means of distribution; and
- Human resources, infrastructure, and confidentiality.

53. Control programs should be designed to include the following elements but not limited to:

- *Inspection, verification, and audit including on-site visits;*
- *Market surveillance;*
- *Sampling and analysis;*
- *Examination of written and other records;*
- *Documentation of observations and of findings; and*
- *Examination of the results of any verification systems operated by the establishment [51].*

As long ago as 1978, in its Report Of The Twelfth Session Of The Codex Committee On Food Labelling Ottawa, May 16–20, 1977, the commission called out such issues as labeling, drained weights, quantitative declarations of ingredients, lot and lot identification, country of origin, date marking, gluten-free foods, claims, and other issues.

Judging from previously cited blatant and more recent food fraud violations, neither governments nor supply chains have established adequate preventive controls.

6.3 GET TRAINING AND GET INVOLVED

Requirements for food safety changes are in a state of relative infancy and while food fraud has been around for many years, beginning to get involved with the prevention of food fraud requires an increase in knowledge. Companies are recommended to search for or develop internal training programs focused on bringing management and all personnel up to a level of understanding and prevention that will enable them to systematically design and implement changes of a preventive nature.

As food supply chains continue to lengthen and become more complex, the potential for food fraud is on the increase. While current publicity tends to focus on illegal substitution issues, standards, labeling, supplier due diligence, packaging, testing, software, and personnel qualification, all need to be addressed. Most management food safety certification programs require management involvement and leadership. Considering that FDA FSMA rules for economically motivated adulteration and the fact that a legal definition of food fraud under the food safety umbrella are yet to be developed, one can be assured that more legal challenges are on the horizon. Regardless of enforcement efforts, protecting one's own brand name and reputation should be of paramount importance to any company.

Establishing a preventive training program for all employees is a must.

6.4 ESTABLISH PREVENTIVE PURCHASING PRACTICES

Purchasing groups need to identify, qualify, certify, and buy only from companies with a strong preventive system in place. If purchasing decisions are based primarily on cost without adequate quality and food safety controls, fraudulent products and ingredients will enter the organization's supply chain and external failures are sure to occur. Preventive programs reduce risk.

Drive ingredient testing and certification down to the supply chain level. As a normal course of business, suppliers must be able to certify the ingredients a company buys along with the practices used to produce or process them. However, depending only on certification has often been shown to be a mistake. Suppliers change personnel and leadership. An approach which requires continuous cooperation and open communication between suppliers and customers goes a long way to preventing misunderstandings and short cuts implemented to deliver against unreasonable schedules and enables preventive thinking and action within the supplier base. A single missed process control at a single supplier should cause that supplier to be able to isolate and correct a product prior to shipment to a customer without the customer having to find or invent a new test capable of discovering the problem.

Expand the thinking that testing of incoming ingredients will solve food fraud problems. Both test technologies and test strategies continue to lag their abilities to detect substituted ingredients and products. Test standards and test requirements should be established between the receiver and the shipper with shipment tests conforming to the receiver's requirements.

6.5 KNOW YOUR SUPPLY CHAIN

An emphasis on knowing the company's supply chain is critical. The idea that one-up and one-down traceability is out of date, especially in light of vicarious liability and newly evolving laws. In the US and across the EU, the interdependence between and among shippers, carriers, and receivers are coming to be viewed in a different light. Knowing that food fraud can enter the supply chain at many distribution points means that a shift from an emphasis on delivery costs and time schedules needs to happen.

Supply chain visibility through chain of custody that includes many levels of traceability in combination with temperature and sanitation monitoring and procedures helps to assure that any receiver can quickly identify and manage suppliers and carriers more interested in saving money than food safety and quality.

In their August 2014 report, the Council of Supply Chain Management Professionals (CSCMP) listed the following food and beverage logistics issues:

1. Food safety
   a. On-time delivery
   b. Traceability
   c. Temperature Abuse
   d. Sabotage and tampering
   e. Contamination
   f. Theft
2. Availability of transport equipment
   a. Reefers
   b. Farm gondolas
   c. Intermodal
   d. Local customers
3. Sustainability of the supply chain
   a. Carbon reduction
   b. Packaging

In that report, the CSCMP noted that "Food safety is the biggest issue and the hardest to get a handle on."

6.6 ESTABLISH A SYSTEM OF DISTRIBUTED AUTHORITY

A system that allows and encourages employees to assume and work beyond imposed organizational authority provides strong employee control and commitment. Conversely, when employees feel they have only responsibility to get the job done, keep their mouths shut, and not rock the boat, they are functioning under authoritarian controls and will not be disposed to identify and report fraudulent ingredients, products, or practices. Placing responsibility on employees without delegating authority is counterproductive and reduces employee honesty, participation, and organizational loyalty.

6.7 INVEST IN PREVENTION BY ESTABLISHING A SYSTEM OF CONTINUOUS IMPROVEMENT

When management assumes a position of good is good enough or "if it ain't broke, don't fix it," efforts to improve systems and practices cease. Operational costs, risk, and the opportunity for escapes go up as does the likelihood of increased costs that open the door for food fraud when continuous improvement systems are sidelined.

Training all employees in food fraud and the opportunities that exist for intentional and unintentional food fraud to enter an organization's system can be greatly reduced by employees who are rewarded for exercising authority along with responsibility, and who are working in a supported continuous improvement atmosphere.

The National Science Foundation (NSF) reports that most food fraud is reported by whistleblowers [52].

Most of these whistleblowers are internal employees working in a corporate culture that might have established less than honest business practices while others work for companies where continuous improvement systems have been established.

6.8 HIRE HONEST PEOPLE

Fraud is often perpetrated by dishonest people. Separating intentional food fraud from unintentional food fraud is a matter that enforcement agencies and courts will later decide. As the earlier Sysco example illustrates, whether intentional or not, food fraud is often the result of some breakdown within the balance between different organizational functions that allow one function to ride herd over less powerful groups. Hiring mature and honest personnel and providing committed leadership and dedicated managerial oversight should become a prime responsibility of the human resources function. While hiring honest personnel is generally a requirement for human resource groups, food fraud requires focus and attention.

6.9 PROACTIVELY COOPERATE WITH THE COMPETITION

Working cooperatively with competitors to prevent food fraud is a preventive approach that is accomplished through associations and organizations. Let's face it, within any industry people move freely from job to job. While there may be competition, there is no way to prevent employees from accepting promotions and raises from a company's competition. Along with the employee go company secrets. Working within established food organizations (e.g., National Fisheries Institute, and the Grocery Manufacturer's Association (GMA)), provides members with knowledge about food fraud, resources, helps all to share preventive tactics, and helps the entire community to protect not only the industry but their own brand names as well. Gathering and sharing food fraud information within and across company boundaries enables the food industry to establish controls and solutions not available to a single company. Sharing food fraud information and solutions is a preventive strategy.

As an example, in June 2015, Seafood Compliance and Labeling Enforcement (SCALE) has been recognized by the US Department of Health and Human Services (HHS) for its training and DNA testing work as part of the FDA's "ongoing integration of forensic science as a way of combating seafood fraud and mislabeling" [53].

With 70–90% of the US seafood supply coming from countries other than the United States, the SCALE approach (Table 6.1 below) has established a comprehensive 2 year plan to tackle seafood fraud [54].

The FDA SCALE project is initially focused on labeling and supply chain issues to determine what type and where violations may be coming from. Reducing the risk of various fish related hazards, such as allergens and toxins, is considered critical to managing the seafood supply chain. The project also illustrates multiagency cooperation with

Table 6.1 SCALE Milestones

A. Develop a regulatory genetic method to identify processed fish filets
B. Build a reference library of DNA sequences for commercial fish
C. With ORA, equip, train, and proficiency test multiple FDA regional field laboratories in fish identification methodology
D. Develop an on-line repository for Standard Operating Procedures (SOPs) and for DNA species reference data for full transparency with other regulatory agencies and industry
E. Make this on-line repository cross-talk with FDA public resources for proper seafood labeling such as the Seafood List: FDA's Guide to Acceptable Market Names for Seafood Sold in Interstate Commerce
F. In conjunction with OFS, OC, and ORA, perform targeted field sampling assignments for high risk species to assess where in the supply chain mislabeling is occurring
G. Develop multi-laboratory validation protocol for fish and crustaceans identification method for submission to FDA Chemical Methods Validation Committee [1]
H. Perform an inter-agency, multi-laboratory validation of fish and crustaceans identification method [1]
I. Develop a regulatory genetic method to identify crab and lobster products
J. Build a reference library for commercial crab and lobster species and add to on-line seafood identification repository
K. Develop SOPs, train regional FDA field laboratories and perform proficiency testing in crab and lobster identification methods
L. Develop a genetic method to identify shrimp products
M. Build a reference library for commercial shrimp species and add to on-line seafood identification repository
N. Develop SOPs, train regional FDA field laboratories and perform proficiency testing in shrimp identification method

involvement of the Office of Food Safety (OFS) Office of Compliance, (OC) and Office of Regulatory Affairs (ORA).

6.10 HELP PROSECUTE AND PUBLICIZE

The discovery of fraudulent food producing, processing, packing, labeling, distributing, or transporting practices within a supply chain harms the entire food chain. Recalls impact everyone and the reputations of the innocent go downhill along with the guilty. Sales also go downhill.

Taking a strong public position in favor of removing the guilty from the system signifies unity among supply chain members and helps to convince suppliers and the consuming public that such practices are not acceptable. The thinking among suppliers that the risk of discovery for shipping fraudulent product is lower than the potential reward if the fraud is not discovered will diminish.

In the EU, many countries (as a result of the horsemeat scandal) are forming their own crime units. With over 3,800 food fraud incidents reported throughout the EU, the Food Standards Agency appointed a new head of the Food Crime Unit [55].

In February 2015, The Herald Scotland published an article stating that Scotland would establish its own crime unit as a result of cumin contaminated with nuts, the horsemeat scandal, counterfeit alcohol, and numerous other violations.

The article reported numerous violations discovered in a worldwide operation in which Interpol cooperated. Some findings included "rotting seafood being sprayed with chemicals and sold as fresh fish, a factory producing fake tea, an unlicensed water bottling plant and fake smoked mozzarella made from out-of-date dairy produce being 'smoked' over burning rubbish" and an "illicit factory in Derbyshire producing fake-name brand vodka using antifreeze" [56].

The National Fisheries Institute (NFI) focuses on seafood fraud through its Better Seafood Board. The Board represents the industry on seafood fraud issues and promotes awareness of seafood fraud, encourages enforcement and awareness of regulations. Lisa Weddig of the Board listed the following issues as of primary concern in a July 2014 presentation:

1. Substitution
2. Inaccurate Country of Origin and wild versus farm labels
3. Selling previously frozen fish as fresh fish
4. And, what they call "qualifiers" including
   a. All natural
   b. Chemical-free
   c. Day boat
   d. Hood and line
   e. Local catch.

Lisa notes that research findings from Boston, Los Angeles, Southern Florida, and Monterey, California show continuing research fraud practices in those regions [57].

CHAPTER 7

Available Resources

At this stage, some individuals and organizations have identified food fraud as an expanding field of study in need of improved controls. While general resources might seem to be lacking at many government levels, others are stepping forward to begin the long search for more comprehensive solutions.

7.1 SOME INTERNATIONAL EXPERTS

Dr Chris Elliott is an analytical chemist and director of the Institute for Global Food Security at Queen's University Belfast, Northern Ireland. In July 2014, he published the "Elliott Review into the Integrity and Assurance of Food Supply Networks—Final Report" which was commissioned by the Secretaries of State for Environment, Food and Rural Affairs, and for Health due to the fraudulent distribution of horse meat throughout the EU.

The report makes several recommendations for food fraud prevention:

1. Protection of consumers is a priority
2. Set zero tolerance as the standard
3. Gather intelligence
4. Provide laboratory services to support audit, inspection, and enforcement
5. Provide audits
6. Improve government support
7. Establish governmental leadership
8. Manage crises through an organized and coordinated system [60].

Dr Elliott also specializes in testing for dioxins, mass spectrometry molecules are converted into ions that can be sorted and measured according to shape and change, DNA testing, PCR, liquid

Food Fraud. DOI: http://dx.doi.org/10.1016/B978-0-12-803393-7.00007-X

chromatography mass spectrometry, and fingerprinting (infrared scanner). He is a strong supporter of mapping the supply chain and moving away from the "one-up and one-back" approach to food safety [61].

Liz Moran is the president of the Association of Public Analysts (APA) in the United Kingdom and is considered a leading food fraud scientist. She has been recognized as one of the top scientists by The UK Science Council.

Dr John Spink (Michigan State University) is perhaps the most well-known food fraud expert in the United States. He has been working on food fraud issues since before 2007 and focuses on anticounterfeiting, packaging, labeling, public policy development, regulatory compliance, risk assessment, economically motivated adulteration, and related issues. Dr Spink has extensive publications in the Journal of Food Protection, Food Technology, Journal of Food Science, the Crime Science Journal and others [62].

Under Dr Spink's Direction, the University of Michigan has established what they call the "Food Fraud Initiative" and offers a number of courses including Food Fraud Overview, Food Fraud Basics, Quantifying Food Fraud Risk, and others. The courses are offered to help companies establish systems for managing food fraud within the industry [63].

Dr Douglas C. Moyer is an associate professor and public health instructor for the University of Michigan specializing in packaging and has been a member of the ISO technical committee TC 247 on food countermeasures and controls. He has recently coauthored and published "Introducing Food Fraud including translation and interpretation to Russian, Korean, and Chinese languages." This work takes a look at preventing food fraud throughout the food chain [64].

There are also a number of local food fraud consultants available to help in different industries. Maureen Downey (WineFraud.com) at Chai Consulting specializes in helping companies to manage their wine inventories and provides wine fraud consulting in the San Francisco Bay area through due diligence practices and training [65].

One fraudster, Rudy Kurnaiwan, specialized in old wine bottles, fake labels, refilling bottles with blends of newer wines, and selling them as rare finds. Rudy was adept at defrauding collectors of rare and very expensive vintages. After receiving a 10-year sentence in the Manhattan federal court, Rudy's defense attorney stated that "Nobody died. Nobody lost their savings. Nobody lost their job."

On April 4, 2015, Karen Stabiner of The New York Times published an article entitled "Private Eyes in the Grocery Aisles," that focused on Mansour Samadpour who is the chief executive officer at IEH Laboratories and Consulting Group. With Costco as a client, IEH tests hundreds of products in their lab. Testing for Costco products is paid for by suppliers—DNA testing costs about $100 per sample tested [66].

7.2 BETTER SEAFOOD BOARD (BSB)

The purpose of the BSB is to educate buyers at the processor, distributor, retail, and restaurant levels of situations of economic fraud in the industry, to highlight companies that have committed to following the rules, and to call-out violators of the rules.

Food Fraud Resources (National Center for Food Protection and Defense)—publications [67].

7.3 FDA DNA SEAFOOD LABELING TRAINING

The FDA established a three part training video to assist seafood personnel and regulators to "ensure the proper labeling of seafood products offered for sale in the US marketplace." The videos can be found at [68].

7.4 FDA FISH SUBSTITUTES

The FDA has also established a list of commonly substituted species of fish. For instance, instead of receiving mahi mahi on your dinner plate, you might be eating yellow tail tuna. Yellow tail is a much cheaper cut of fish than mahi mahi and price cuts are a common reason for fish substitution [69].

Barfblog (safe food from farm to fork) lists numerous interesting examples of food fraud practices [70].

7.5 THE UNIVERSITY OF MICHIGAN FOOD FRAUD INITIATIVE

The University of Michigan Food Fraud Initiative provides a number of food fraud training courses including food fraud basics, food fraud overview, quantifying food risk, food fraud trends, food defense strategy, and others. The Initiative states its mission is "to leverage Michigan State University's broad leadership position to protect the global and domestic food supply from Food Fraud vulnerability" [71].

7.6 THE US PHARMACOPEIAL FOOD FRAUD DATABASE

The USP Food Fraud Database is located at [72] and provides food fraud searches and a report mechanism.

7.7 FOOD FRAUDSTER

Under the auspices of the National Food Protection Collaboratory, Food Fraudster represents itself as a "computing tool specific to identifying and mitigating food fraud concerns within the food industry." Food Fraudster covers country of origin, the production chain, monitoring of incidents, countermeasures, alerts, and food fraud assessments. Membership prices range from $100 per year for alerts to $11,400 per year for entire coverage for a retailer [73].

7.8 UK FOOD STANDARDS AGENCY "REPORTING FOOD FRAUD"

The UK Food standards Agency provides a food fraud search option and information related to the National Food Crime Unit, whistle-blowing, recycling, packaging, "use by" dates, the Food Fraud Advisory Unit, food alerts, and other information [74].

7.9 EUROPEAN COMMISSION OFFICIAL CONTROLS AND ENFORCEMENT

The European Commission provides information related to the food fraud 5-point action plan, the network of food fraud contacts and other relevant information [75].

7.10 NATIONAL CENTER FOR FOOD PROTECTION AND DEFENSE: FOOD FRAUD RESOURCES

Food Fraud Resources provides a series of food fraud publication available to the public. The publications cover topics such as economically motivated adulteration, "current technologies for the detection of food adulteration and contamination," a database focused on food fraud, deterrence and detection, seafood fraud, and others [76].

7.11 NATIONAL SCIENCE FOUNDATION (NSF)

NSF provides market intelligence, expert and specialist consulting, training, help with supplier selection, information on traceability, references to laboratory testing facilities, and information on certification programs. NSF also publishes relevant information on "Food Fraud Awareness, Detection & Prevention" [77].

7.12 RAPID ALERT SYSTEM FOR FOOD AND FEED (RASFF)

Software may provide the opportunity for many companies to proactively identify problem suppliers prior to purchase. The Rapid Alert System for Food and Feed (RASFF) database established by the EU provides feed and food safety alerts of all kinds. Access to the RASFF portal provides businesses, consumers, government agencies, and others with the ability to search the database by product, keyword, date, hazard, country, and whether or not the product was in the distribution system [58,60].

Perkin Elmer provides "New Adulterant Screen" software that provides a rapid "pass/fail screening for adulterants" to help authenticate ingredients [59].

Sciex (Sciex.com) provides software enabled equipment including capillary, electrophoresis, ion mobility spectrometry, mass spectrometers, and other solutions for food fraud screening.

CHAPTER 8

Summary: Confusion Reigns

Food fraud and the potential for food fraud come from many more directions than mere substitution of one product or ingredient for another. And food fraud is practiced at many levels from the restaurant waitress telling customers that tilapia is cod to the blatant replacement of beef with horse meat, and the use of contaminated packing materials in order to save money. While food fraud has been around since time began and is costing billions of dollars each year on a world-wide basis, the drive to bring things under some semblance of control is in its infancy.

The entire supply chain is called to task to begin to work on assessments and plans focused on risk reduction and preventive planning and to work collectively to establish a chain of custody system.

On the negative side, the lack of unified legal definitions, governmental leadership, labeling and packaging standards, food fraud reporting, low cost rapid test strategies, competent resources and specialists, cooperation among competitors, uniform prosecution, ability to hire personnel capable of making honest decisions, supply chain traceability and monitoring, knowledge and implementation of preventive purchasing practices, training and commitment all combine to paint a dismal picture when it comes to reducing food fraud risk and prevention.

While protecting brand integrity might motivate a processor or the Grocery Manufacturers Association (GMA) to prevent food fraud, their ability to improve product safety and establish preventive practices is seriously lacking. The food supply chain is in a reactive mode and the movement from reaction to preventive strategy is likely to take a generation of effort from all supply chain members. Needed changes are progressing on many fronts, but due to a lack of appropriate and unifying laws (other than interstate transportation regulations), enforcement is haphazard.

Food Fraud. DOI: http://dx.doi.org/10.1016/B978-0-12-803393-7.00008-1

Requirements for systematized traceability systems can be seen as a key component to prevention. In many industries, chain of custody requirements serve not only to assure product traceability but to establish a means to enforcement. While food supply chains and governments continue to resist defining basic traceability standards at the unit, case, pallet, or container levels, recall of impacted product can take weeks or months. The long search for causes that often accompany recall efforts fuel industry and consumer fears and destroy clean markets along with those intentionally or unknowingly involved in fraudulent practices.

Although scattered and often confused, international resources are slowly becoming available to help define, train, and implement preventive, risk reducing solutions. The technology capable of delivering accurate and timely test solutions is quickly evolving in support of supplier ingredient final product testing. The cost and effectiveness of cell phone based temperature monitoring solutions are ever improving due to demand and market competiveness. While sometimes the refusal to improve and modernize packaging and packaging practices can be seen as an economic motivator to adulteration, current food safety requirements call for changes in package production, storage, and handling that will provide known protection for product in contact with package interior surfaces.

In spite of adequate regulation and governmental guidance, label issues continue to dominate the food fraud and recall arenas. Food companies often collectively cooperate to resist consumer and governmental efforts to require, change, and enforce label standards designed to eliminate deception and provide improved informed consumer decision making.

At times, the food safety system itself needs to be called into question as government officials intentionally withhold information critical to driving recognition of food fraud problems and systematic change. There is occasional evidence regarding the inadequacy and incompleteness of food safety audits that either do not know how to control the quality of their efforts or do not want to confront issues. A company that passes a food safety audit 1 day and causes illness and death the next day clearly indicates there are problems within the food safety system.

Recommendations designed to establish a prevention driving chain of custody approach to many food fraud issues would call for taking a responsible and involved approach that involves hiring, training, and managing all employees in a different manner, working cooperatively across industry boundaries and helping to identify and rid the food industry of food fraudsters and fraudulent food practices.

REFERENCES

[1] Webster's ninth new collegiate dictionary, Merriam-Webster Inc., Springfield, MA, 111983.

[2] September 21, 2014 <http://www.cnn.com/2014/09/19/us/peanut-butter-salmonella-trial/>.

[3] October 31, 2013 <http://www.foodsafetynews.com/2013/10/jensen-brothers-sue-primus-over-third-party-audit-they-say-was-faulty/#.Vb-B8flLXZk>.

[4] July 28, 2015 <http://www.gmaonline.org/downloads/wygwam/consumerproductfraud.pdf>.

[5] Johnson R, <http://fas.org/sgp/crs/misc/R43358.pdf> – May 2015 Food fraud and "Economically Motivated Adulteration" of food and food ingredients, Renée Johnson, Specialist in Agricultural Policy, January 10, 2014.

[6] Federal Register 64: 15497–15499, April 6, 2009.

[7] May 3, 2014 <http://www.theguardian.com/world/2014/feb/07/fake-food-scandal-revealed-tests-products-mislabelled>.

[8] July 16, 2015 <https://www.food.gov.uk/enforcement/foodfraud>.

[9] June 1, 2015 <http://ec.europa.eu/food/safety/official_controls/food_fraud/index_en.htm>.

[10] August 1, 2015 <http://foodfraud.msu.edu/wp-content/uploads/2014/07/food-fraud-ffg-back-grounder-v11-Final.pdf>.

[11] July 25, 2015 <http://www.regulations.gov/#%21docketDetail;D=FDA-2013-N-1425>.

[12] August 13, 2015 <https://www.federalregister.gov/articles/2013/12/24/2013-30373/focused-mitigation-strategies-to-protect-food-against-intentional-adulteration>.

[13] July 21, 2015 <http://www.fda.gov/ICECI/ComplianceManuals/RegulatoryProceduresManual/ucm176738.htm>.

[14] Moore JC, Spink J, Lipp M. Development and application of a database of food ingredient fraud and economically motivated adulteration from 1980 to 2010. J Food Sci 2012;77(4): and USP, Food Fraud Database, Glossary of Terms.

[15] June 13, 2015 <http://www.justice.gov/usam/civil-resource-manual-120-sample-indictment-food-fraud-prosecution-miscellaneous-counts>.

[16] July 21, 2015 <https://www.wklaw.com/distributing-mislabeled-products-in-interstate-com-merce/>.

[17] July 21, 2015, Lanza EM, pp5 Food safety issues: FDA judicial enforcement actions, Legislative Attorney, March 3, 2015 <http://nationalaglawcenter.org/wp-content/uploads/assets/crs/R43927.pdf>.

[18] May 13, 2015 <http://www.fda.gov/Food/GuidanceRegulation/GuidanceDocumentsRegulatory Information/LabelingNutrition/ucm064866.htm>.

[19] July 21, 22015 <http://www.foodsafety.gov/recalls/recent/index.html>.

[20] July 2, 2015 <https://webgate.ec.europa.eu/rasff-window/portal/?event=searchResultList>.

[21] May 15, 2015, Full text: China's food quality and safety, August 17, 2007 <http://www.gov.cn/english/2007-08/17/content_720346.htm>.

[22] July 15, 2014 <http://www.foodsafetynews.com/2014/07/study-175-hazardous-chemicals-legally-used-to-produce-food-packaging/#.VaerL_lLXZk>

[23] Geueke B, Wagner CC, Muncke J. Food contact substances and chemicals of concern: a comparison of inventories. Food Addit Contam, A 2014; July 7, 2014 <http://www.tandfonline.com/doi/abs/10.1080/19440049.2014.931600?journalCode=tfac20>

[24] April 5, 2015 <http://www.astm.org/Standards/paper-and-packaging-standards.html>.

[25] June 26, 2015 <http://www.fda.gov/AJAX/All/default.htm?Label=All+Recalls>.

[26] June 26, 2016 <http://ec.europa.eu/food/fs/sc/scf/out112_en.pdf>.

[27] June 26, 2015 <http://www.foodproductiondaily.com/Processing/FDA-asked-to-rescind-use-of-carbon-monoxide-for-meats>.

[28] July 10, 2015 Pepsi's "Aquafina" bottled water, is tap water, Mercola.com, <http://articles.mercola.com/sites/articles/archive/2007/08/16/pepsi-s-aquafina-bottled-water-is-tap-water.aspx>.

[29] August 6, 2015 <http://www.fda.gov/Food/FoodborneIllnessContaminants/BuyStoreServe SafeFood/ucm077079.htm>.

[30] August 6, 2015 <http://www.accessdata.fda.gov/scripts/cdrh/cfdocs/cfcfr/CFRSearch.cfm? fr=101.18>.

[31] Lalumandier JA, Ayers LW. Fluoride and bacterial content of bottled water vs tap water. Arch Fam Med 2000;9(3):246–50.

[32] August 7, 2015 <http://well.blogs.nytimes.com/2015/02/03/new-york-attorney-general-targets-supplements-at-major-retailers/?_r=0>.

[33] Newmaster SG, Grguric M, Shanmughanandhan D, Ramalingam S, Ragupathy S. DNA barcoding detects contamination and substitution in North American herbal products. BMC Med 2013;11:222 August 6, 2015 http://dx.doi.org/10.1186/1741-7015-11-222. Published: 11 October 2013

[34] August 7, 2015 <https://www.consumerlab.com/recalls.asp>.

[35] June 2, 2015 <http://www.freightwatchintl.com>.

[36] April 15, 2015 <http://www.fda.gov/ICECI/CriminalInvestigations/ucm209979.htm>.

[37] July 29, 2015 <http://www.bloomberg.com/bw/articles/2013-09-19/how-germany-s-alw-got-busted-for-the-largest-food-fraud-in-u-dot-s-dot-history>.

[38] August 3, 2015 <http://www.foodfraud.org/search/site>.

[39] August 3, 2015 <http://www.tandfonline.com/doi/abs/10.1080/10408690590956369>.

[40] July 13, 2015 <http://www.forbes.com/sites/bethhoffman/2013/10/23/top-10-at-risk-fraudulent-foods-surprising-and-disheartening/>.

[41] July 16, 2015 <http://www.nbcbayarea.com/news/local/Sysco-Food-Stored-in-Dirty-Sheds-Served-to-Bay-Area-Restaurants-215759351.html>.

[42] November 13, 2014 <http://www.nbcbayarea.com/investigations/Sysco-Fined-Millions-for-Storing-Seafood-Milk-and-Raw-Meat-in-Unrefrigerated-Sheds-267554391.html>.

[43] November 12, 2014 <http://media.nbcbayarea.com/documents/sysco_final_narrative_signed_scanned_Redacted.pdf>.

[44] July 27, 2015 <http://www.sysco.com/customer-solutions/high-tech-tools-for-fighting-food-fraud.html>.

[45] Feb 30, 2015 <http://www.latimes.com/food/dailydish/la-dd-kraft-recall-american-cheese-sin-gles-20140902-story.html>.

[46] August 5, 2015 <http://articles.mercola.com/sites/articles/archive/2013/05/04/food-fraud.aspx>.

[47] July 1, 2015 <http://www.ift.org/gftc.aspx>.

[48] July 22, 2015 <http://www.today.com/id/48691046/ns/today-today_news/t/rossen-reports-some-trucks-carry-unsafe-food-authorities-say/#.Va-04PlLXZk>.

[49] Webster's new world law dictionary, Copyright © 2010, Wiley Publishing, Inc., Hoboken, NJ.

[50] August 10, 2015 <https://en.wikipedia.org/wiki/Chain_of_custody>.

[51] July 29, 2015, Principles and guidelines for national food control systems CAC/GL 82-2013.

[52] July 26, 2015 <http://www.nsf.org/newsroom_pdf/NSF_Food_Fraud_Whitepaper.pdf)>.

[53] July 26, 2015 <https://www.aboutseafood.com/category/overall-taxonomy/better-seafood-bureau>.

[54] July 27, 2015 <http://www.accessdata.fda.gov/scripts/fdatrack/view/track_project.cfm?program=cfsan&id=CFSAN-ORS-Fish-Scale>.

[55] May 15, 2015 <https://www.food.gov.uk/news-updates/news/2015/13743/new-head-of-the-food-crime-unit>.

[56] July 21, 2015 <http://www.heraldscotland.com/news/13202739.Scotland_gets_its_own_crime_unit_to_fight_food_fraud/>.

[57] July 25, 2015 – May 3, 2014 Presentation by Lisa Weddig, NFI, <http://www.foodprotect.org/media/meeting/2014%20CFP%20Seafood%20Fraud%20Presentation%20LWeddig.pdf>.

[58] July 27, 2015 <https://webgate.ec.europa.eu/rasffwindow/portal/?event=SearchForm&cleanSearch=1>.

[59] July 27, 2015 <http://www.perkinelmer.com/industries/food-beverage-nutraceuticals/food-fraud.xhtml>.

[60] Elliott review into the integrity and assurance of food supply networks – final report. Crown copyright 2014, <https://www.gov.uk/government/uploads/system/uploads/attachment_data/file/350726/elliot-review-final-report-july2014.pdf>.

[61] July 13, 2015 <http://futurefood2050.com/arresting-food-fraud/>. – Future Food 2050 – Arresting Food Fraud [accessed 3.18.15].

[62] June 15, 2015 <http://foodfraud.msu.edu/wp-content/uploads/2015/01/biosketch-nih-format-cv-spink-jws-2014-12-16.pdf>.

[63] July 24, 2015 <http://foodfraud.msu.edu/>.

[64] Spink J, Moyer DC, Park H, Wu Y, Fersht V, Shao B, et al. Food Chem 2015;189:102–7 Epub 2014 Sep 28

[65] July 27, 2015 <http://www.chaiconsulting.com>.

[66] July 15, 2015 <http://www.nytimes.com/2015/04/05/business/private-eyes-in-the-grocery-aisles.html?_r=0>.

[67] June 10 2015 <http://www.foodfraudresources.com/publications/>.

[68] August 4, 2015 <http://www.fda.gov/Food/GuidanceRegulation/GuidanceDocumentsRegulatoryInformation/Seafood/ucm419982.htm>.

[69] August 4, 2015 <http://www.fda.gov/Food/FoodScienceResearch/RFE/ucm071528.htm>.

[70] July 15, 2015 <http://barfblog.com/tags/food-fraud/>.

[71] August 4, 2015 <http://foodfraud.msu.edu/2013/02/20/introducing-the-food-fraud-initiative-and-mooc/>.

[72] July 21, 2015 <http://www.usp.org/food-ingredients/food-fraud-database>.

[73] April 15, 2015 <http://nfpcportal.com/FQTools/FoodFraudster/tabid/329/Default.aspx>.

[74] August 3, 2015 <https://www.food.gov.uk/enforcement/the-national-food-crime-unit/foodfraud>.

[75] August 4, 2015 <http://ec.europa.eu/food/safety/official_controls/food_fraud/index_en.htm>.

[76] August 1, 2015 <http://www.foodfraudresources.com/publications/>.

[77] July 11, 2015 <http://www.nsf.org/services/by-industry/food-safety-quality/food-fraud/>.

Printed in the United States
by Baker & Taylor Publisher Services